McGraw-Hill Education

Nursing
Spanish
Visual
Phrasebook

Neil Bobenhouse, MHA, EMT-P
with Dean Meenach, RN, BSN, CEN, CCRN

New York Chicago San Francisco Athens London Madrid
Mexico City Milan New Delhi Singapore Sydney Toronto

1 2 3 4 5 6 7 8 9 10 CTP/CTP 1 0 9 8 7 6 5 4 3

ISBN   978-0-07-180890-3
MHID   0-07-180890-6

e-ISBN   978-0-07-180891-0
e-MHID   0-07-180891-4

Library of Congress Control Number 2013930338

NOTICE

This book is not intended to provide medical advice or to substitute for the advice of a licensed medical professional, and readers should consult an appropriate medical practitioner for all matters relating to their health. Medicine is an ever-changing science. As new research and clinical experience broaden our knowledge, changes in treatment and drug therapy are required. The authors and the publisher of this work have checked with sources believed to be reliable in their efforts to provide information that is complete and generally in accord with the standards accepted at the time of publication. However, in view of the possibility of human error or changes in medical sciences, neither the authors nor the publisher nor any other party who has been involved in the preparation or publication of this work warrants that the information contained herein is in every respect accurate or complete, and they disclaim all responsibility for any errors or omissions or for the results obtained from use of the information contained in this work. Readers are encouraged to confirm the information contained herein with other sources. For example and in particular, readers are advised to check the product information sheet included in the package of each drug they plan to administer to be certain that any information contained in this work is accurate and that changes have not been made in the recommended dose or in the contraindications for administration.

Credits appear on page 152

McGraw-Hill Education products are available at special quantity discounts to use as premiums and sales promotions or for use in corporate training programs. To contact a representative, please visit the Contact Us pages at www.mhprofessional.com.

This book is printed on acid-free paper.

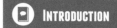

ABOUT THE PHRASEBOOK

McGraw-Hill Education's Nursing Spanish Visual Phrasebook is a communication aid specifically designed for EMTs, paramedics, nurses, physicians, and other healthcare providers who need to communicate with non-English-speaking patients. This book is a valuable bridge for healthcare providers to better understand their patients before proper translation services can be accessed. You do not need to know any language other than English to successfully use this book. All foreign language elements are presented with visual images or phrased as yes-no questions. Non-English speaking patients can point to the relevant images or respond to simple questions with a nod of the head or a simple "yes" or "no" in order to communicate essential information. The book is designed to be useful from intake to discharge. Primary assessments ask general questions while the secondary assessments contain in-depth questions for specific specialties. These assessments feature the most basic words and phrases that allow you to get essential information from patients. Secondary assessments are divided into three sections: Acute History, Procedural, and Past History. Procedural sections contain statements that may be useful when examining a patient or communicating what might be happening.

As with any medical assessment, a subjective account must be considered with vital signs and other objective measures. THIS PHRASEBOOK IS NOT A DIAGNOSTIC DEVICE AND CANNOT DIAGNOSE MEDICAL CONDITIONS. THIS PHRASEBOOK IS STRICTLY A TRANSLATION AID. It must be understood that no translation is absolute and perfect. All translations were written with a general audience in mind.

HOW TO USE THIS PHRASEBOOK

The sequence of questions is intended to flow with a normal assessment but written to be stand alone questions as well. Questions were ordered from "head to toe," "onset, provocation, quality, radiation, strength, time," and increasing focus. Secondary Assessment sections were focused on immediate signs/symptoms, procedures that would begin shortly after, and long-term history. This general format is amended in certain areas as needed.

Contents

CONTENTS

Secondary Assessment and History

CONTENTS

SECONDARY ASSESSMENT AND HISTORY (CONTINUED)

SECONDARY PROCEDURAL

CONTENTS

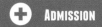
Hola, soy un(a) profesional de la salud. No hablo español.
Hello, I am a healthcare professional. I do not speak Spanish.

Respóndame solo sí no o no lo sé .
Respond to me "yes," "no" or "I don't know."

¿Está usted aquí por un problema médico o de enfermedad?

Are you here for a medical problem or sickness?

¿Está usted aquí debido a una lesión física?

Are you here because of a physical injury?

Por favor, anote su nombre claramente.
Please write your name clearly.

_____

Por favor, anote la fecha actual claramente.
Please write the current date clearly.

____ / ____ / ____
DÍA   MES   AÑO

Por favor, anote su dirección de correo claramente.
Please write your mailing address clearly.

_____
Calle (Street)   Apartamento (Apt. #)

_____
Ciudad (City)   Estado (State)   Código Postal (ZIP)

DEMOGRAPHICS

2

Por favor, anote su número de teléfono claramente.

Please write your phone number clearly.

(_____) _____ - _____

Por favor, anote su número de seguro social.

Please write your Social Security number.

_____ - _____ - _____

Por favor, permítame su licencia de conducir o identificación Estatal. Tengo que sacarle una copia y se la devolveré en breve.

Please give me your driver's license or State ID. I need to make a copy of it and will return it to you shortly.

¿Tiene seguro médico?

Do you have medical insurance?

Por favor, permítame su tarjeta de seguro. Tengo que sacarle una copia y se la devolveré en breve.

Please give me your insurance card. I need to make a copy of it and will return it to you shortly.

¿Se le considera legalmente hombre o mujer?

Are you legally male or female?

 Hombre
Male

 Mujer
Female

¿Tiene empleo?
Are you employed?

Por favor, anote el nombre del lugar donde trabaja.
Please write the name of your place of work.

Por favor, párese en la báscula.
Please step on this scale.

¿Cuál es su estado civil?
What is your marital status?

 Soltero(a)
Single

 Divorciado(a)
Divorced

 Casado(a)
Married

 Viudo(a)
Widowed

¿Necesita ayuda para bañarse, comer, vestirse o cuidar de su hogar?
Do you need help with bathing, eating, dressing, or taking care of your household?

¿Se encuentra usted en una relación donde corre peligro físico o emocional?
Are you in a harmful physical or emotional relationship?

4

¿Tiene redactado un documento de
instrucciones anticipadas?

Do you have an advanced directive?

¿Bebe más de cinco bebidas alcohólicas al día?

Do you drink more than five alcoholic drinks a day?

 Sí
Yes

 No
No

 Dejé el trago
I quit

Por favor, indique el tipo de bebida alcohólica que normalmente bebe.

Please indicate type of alcohol you normally drink.

 Cerveza
Beer

 Whiskey
Whiskey

 Vodka
Vodka

 Bourbon
Bourbon

Vino
Wine

Otra
Other

 Ginebra
Gin

¿Fuma cigarrillos o utiliza productos de tabaco?

Do you smoke cigarettes or use tobacco products?

 Sí
Yes

 No
No

 Dejé de fumar
I quit

¿Ha tenido un resultado positivo
en la prueba de la tuberculosis?

Have you had a positive test for tuberculosis?

¿Utiliza alguna droga ilícita o medicamentos que no fueron prescritos para usted?

Do you use any illicit drugs/medications that are not prescribed to you?

 Sí
Yes

 No
No

 Dejé las drogas
I quit

Por favor, indique qué tipo de drogas utiliza.

Please indicate what type of drugs you use.

 Cocaína
Cocaine

 Éxtasis
Ecstasy

 Heroína
Heroin

 LSD/ "ácido"
LSD/"acid"

 Marihuana
Marijuana

 Metanfetaminas
Methamphetamines

 Otra
Other

Por favor, indique de qué forma usa estas drogas.

Please indicate in which form you use these drugs.

 Inyectada por
vía intravenosa
Inject intravenously

 Introducida por vía rectal
Insert rectally

 Fumada
Smoke

 Aspirada por la nariz
Snort

 Por vía oral en forma
de píldora
Swallow in pill form

 Otra
Other

¿Usa gafas y/o contactos?
Do you wear glasses and/or contacts?

¿Usa aparatos auditivos?
Do you wear hearing aids?

¿Cómo describiría su apetito?
How would you describe your appetite?

 Normal
Normal

 Anormal
Abnormal

 Inconsistente
Inconsistent

 Más de lo normal
Greater than normal

 Menos de lo normal
Less than normal

¿Cómo describiría su dieta?
How would you describe your diet?

 Saludable
Healthy

 Más o menos saludable
Somewhat healthy

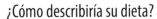 **Ni saludable ni no saludable**
Neither healthy nor unhealthy

 Poco saludable
Somewhat unhealthy

 No saludable
Unhealthy

¿La razón por la cual está aquí está
relacionada con el trabajo?
Is the reason why you are here work related?

MEDICAL ASSESSMENT

Hola, soy un(a) profesional de la salud. No hablo español.

Hello, I am a healthcare professional. I do not speak Spanish.

Respóndame solo sí o no .

Only respond to me "yes" or "no."

¿Actualmente tiene o ha tenido recientemente los siguientes síntomas?

Do you currently have/recently had the following symptoms?

Spanish			English
Dolor abdominal			Abdominal pain
Dolores musculares			Aches
Dolor de espalda			Back pain
Nacidos o abscesos			Boil or abscess
Dolor en los huesos o en las articulaciones			Bone or joint pain
Dolor en el pecho			Chest pain
Escalofríos			Chills
Diarrea			Diarrhea
Dificultad para tragar			Difficulty swallowing
Dificultad para hablar			Difficulty talking
Dificultad para caminar y/o moverse			Difficulty walking/moving
Mareos			Dizziness
Dolor en los oídos			Earache

Spanish			English
Dolor en los ojos	✓	✗	Eye pain
Fiebre	✓	✗	A fever
Dolor en los genitales	✓	✗	Genital pain
Dolor de cabeza	✓	✗	A headache
Problemas de la audición	✓	✗	Hearing problems
Dolor en la pierna	✓	✗	Leg pain
Náuseas	✓	✗	Nausea
Secreción del pezón	✓	✗	Nipple discharge
Entumecimiento u hormigueo	✓	✗	Numbness or tingling
Sangrado nasal	✓	✗	A nose bleed
Erupción	✓	✗	Rash
Sangrado rectal	✓	✗	Rectal bleeding
Falta de aire / dificultad para respirar	✓	✗	Shortness of breath
Dolor en el hombro	✓	✗	Shoulder pain
Cambio de color en la piel	✓	✗	Skin color change
Dolor de garganta	✓	✗	A sore throat
Dolor de estómago	✓	✗	Stomach pain

MEDICAL ASSESSMENT

¿Actualmente tiene o ha tenido recientemente los siguientes síntomas?
Do you currently have/recently had the following symptoms?

Hinchazón	✓	✗	Swelling
Dificultad para orinar	✓	✗	Urination difficulty
Problemas de visión	✓	✗	Vision problems
Vómito	✓	✗	Vomiting
Debilidad	✓	✗	Weakness

¿Los síntomas comenzaron hoy?
Did your symptoms begin today?

Sírvase indicar a qué hora comenzaron los síntomas hoy.
Please indicate what time your symptoms began today.

AM	1	2	3	4	5	6	7	8	9	10	11	12
PM	1	2	3	4	5	6	7	8	9	10	11	12

¿Los síntomas comenzaron esta semana?
Did your symptoms begin this week?

Sírvase indicar cuantos días han pasado desde el inicio de los síntomas.
Please indicate how many days have passed since your symptoms began.

1   2   3   4   5   6   7

MEDICAL ASSESSMENT

10

¿Los síntomas comenzaron hace más de una semana?
Did your symptoms begin longer than a week ago?

Sírvase indicar cuantas semanas han pasado desde el inicio de los síntomas.
Please indicate how many weeks have passed since your symptoms began.

| **SEMANAS** | 1 | 2 | 3 | 4 | 5 | 6 | 7 | 8 | 9 | 10 | > |
| WEEKS | | | | | | | | | | | |

| **MESES** | 1 | 2 | 3 | 4 | 5 | 6 | 7 | 8 | 9 | 10 | > |
| MONTHS | | | | | | | | | | | |

¿Ha experimentado estos síntomas previamente?
Have you experienced these symptoms previously?

¿Tiene estos síntomas varias veces?
Do you have these symptoms repeatedly?

¿Cuándo fue la última vez que tomó sus medicamentos?
When did you last take your prescribed medications?

| **DÍAS** | 1 | 2 | 3 | 4 | 5 | 6 | 7 | > |
| DAYS | | | | | | | | |

¿Cuándo fue la última vez que comió?
When is the last time you had food?

| **DÍAS** | 1 | 2 | 3 | 4 | 5 | 6 | 7 | > |
| DAYS | | | | | | | | |

¿Puede comer alimentos sólidos sin dificultad?
Can you eat solid foods without difficulty?

¿Puede beber líquidos sin dificultad?
Can you drink liquids without difficulty?

PHYSICAL ASSESSMENT

Hola, soy un(a) profesional de la salud. No hablo español.

Hello, I am a healthcare professional. I do not speak Spanish.

Por favor, señale (en este dibujo de una persona) donde tiene dolor.

Please point (on this picture of a person) to where you have pain.

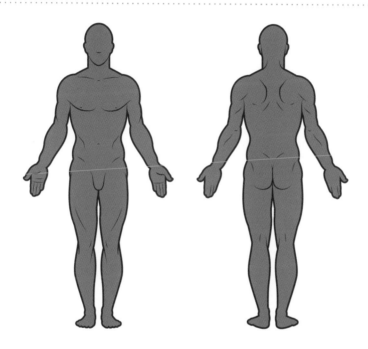

Por favor, indique (en la siguiente escala) la intensidad de su dolor.

Please point (on this scale) to rate your pain.

No hay dolor   Dolor moderado   Dolor intenso

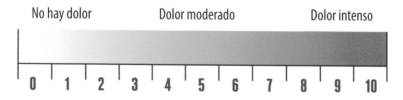

0 1 2 3 4 5 6 7 8 9 10

¿Cuándo ocurrió la lesión?
When did your injury occur?

MINUTOS MINUTES	10	20	30	40	50	60				
HORAS HOURS	2	4	6	8	10	12	14	16	18	20	22
DÍAS DAYS	1	2	3	4	5	6	7	8	9	10	>
MESES MONTHS	1	2	3	4	5	6	7	8	9	10	>
AÑOS YEARS	1	2	3	4	5	6	7	8	9	10	>

¿Qué causó esta lesión?
What caused this injury?

- Fui agredido
  Assault
- Un accidente de vehículo todo terreno o de moto
  ATV/Motorcycle accident
- Un accidente de carro
  Car accident
- Estrujado o apretado
  Crush
- Una caída
  Fall
- Lesiones deportivas
  Sports injury
- Otro
  Other
- No lo sé
  I don't know

¿Perdió el conocimiento?
Did you lose consciousness?

PHYSICAL ASSESSMENT

13

¿Cómo describiría el dolor?
How would you describe your pain?

✓ **Persistente**
Aching

✓ **Insistente**
Nagging

✓ **Abrazador**
Burning

✓ **Agudo**
Sharp

✓ **Devastador**
Crushing

✓ **Fulgurante**
Shooting

✓ **Sordo**
Dull

✓ **Lacerante**
Stabbing

¿Vacunado contra el tétano en los últimos 5 años?
Have you had a tetanus shot within the past 5 years?

¿Cuándo fue la última vez que tomó sus medicamentos?
When did you last take your prescribed medications?

DÍAS   1   2   3   4   5   6   7   >

¿Cuándo fue la última vez que comió?
When is the last time you had food?

DÍAS   1   2   3   4   5   6   7   >

¿Puede comer alimentos sólidos sin dificultad?
Can you eat solid foods without difficulty?

¿Puede beber líquidos sin dificultad?
Can you drink liquids without difficulty?

EXPANDED QUESTIONS

14
ASSAULT

. . . .

¿Con qué lo atacaron?
What were you attacked with?

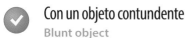 **Con un objeto contundente**
Blunt object

✓ **Otro**
Other

✓ **A puños**
Fist

✓ **No lo sé.**
I don't know.

✓ **Con puñal**
Knife

¿Cuántas veces?
How many times?

1   2   3   4   5   >   ?

ATV/MOTORCYCLE ACCIDENT

. . . .

¿Usted estaba usando casco?
Were you wearing a helmet?

¿Usted fue expulsado de su vehículo?
Were you ejected off your vehicle?

¿Ha tomado bebidas alcohólicas el día de hoy?
Have you been drinking alcohol today?

¿Ha usado drogas recreativas el día de hoy?
Have you been using recreational drugs today?

. . . .

MOTOR VEHICLE CRASH

¿Usted recuerda lo que sucedió?
Do you remember what happened?

¿Usted tenía el cinturón de seguridad abrochado?
Were you wearing a seatbelt?

¿Dónde estaba usted sentado?
Where were you sitting?

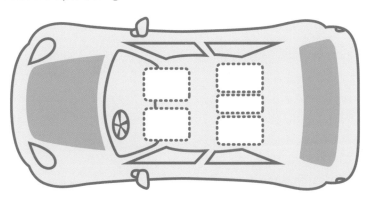

¿Se inflaron las bolsas de aire?
Did your airbags deploy?

¿Tiene entumecimiento u hormigueo en los brazos?
Do you have numbness or tingling in your arms?

¿Tiene debilidad en los brazos?
Do you have weakness in your arms?

¿Tiene entumecimiento u hormigueo en las piernas?
Do you have numbness or tingling in your legs?

¿Tiene debilidad en las piernas?
Do you have weakness in your legs?

¿Perdió el conocimiento?
Did you lose consciousness?

¿Salió del carro por sus propios medios?
Did you get out of the car on your own?

¿Le duele el cuello o espalda?
Does your neck or back hurt?

¿Ha estado tomando alcohol?
Have you been drinking alcohol?

¿Ha estado utilizando drogas ilícitas?
Have you been using illicit drugs?

¿Recuerda lo que pasó antes del accidente?
Do you remember what happened before the crash?

¿Recuerda lo que pasó después del accidente?
Do you remember what happened after the crash?

FALL

¿De qué altura se cayó?
From what height did you fall?

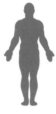

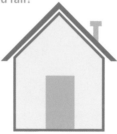

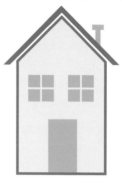

Sentado	De pie	Edificio de 1 piso	Edificio de 2 pisos o más
Sitting	Standing	One story	Two stories or more

¿Se golpeó la cabeza?
Did you hit your head?

¿Perdió el conocimiento?
Did you lose consciousness?

¿Tiene entumecimiento u hormigueo en los brazos?
Do you have numbness or tingling in your arms?

¿Tiene debilidad en los brazos?
Do you have weakness in your arms?

¿Tiene entumecimiento u hormigueo en las piernas?
Do you have numbness or tingling in your legs?

¿Tiene debilidad en las piernas?
Do you have weakness in your legs?

EXPANDED QUESTIONS

18

SPORTS INJURY

¿Qué deporte estaba practicando cuando se lesionó?
What sport were you injured playing?

Fútbol Americano
American Football

Baloncesto
Basketball

Béisbol
Baseball

Fútbol
Soccer

Hockey
Hockey

Tenis
Tennis

Patinaje Sobre Ruedas
Rollerskating

Skateboarding
Skateboarding

Esquí
Skiing

Snowboard
Snowboarding

Levantamiento de Pesas
Weightlifting

Otro
Other

¿Usted estaba usando casco?
Were you wearing a helmet?

¿Estaba usando un suspensorio atlético para los genitales?
Were you wearing an athletic supporter for your genitalia?

¿Perdió el conocimiento?
Did you lose consciousness?

Hola, soy un(a) profesional de la salud. No hablo español.

Hello, I am a healthcare professional. I do not speak Spanish.

Respóndame solo sí no o no lo sé ? .

Respond to me "yes," "no" or "I don't know."

ALLERGIES

¿Tiene alergia a algún medicamento?

Do you have allergies to any medications?

¿Tiene alergia a alguna comida?

Do you have allergies to any foods?

¿Sufre de alergia estacional?

Do you have seasonal allergies?

¿Es usted alérgico al látex?

Are you allergic to latex?

MEDICATIONS

¿Usted toma medicamentos prescritos en casa?

Do you take prescribed medications at home?

¿Tiene sus medicamentos aquí?

Do you have your medications with you?

Por favor, muéstreme sus medicamentos.

Please show me your medications.

Hola, soy un(a) profesional de la salud. No hablo español.

Hello, I am a healthcare professional. I do not speak Spanish.

Respóndame solo sí o no .

Only respond to me "yes" or "no."

PAST MEDICAL HISTORY

¿Usted toma medicamentos prescritos en casa?

Do you take prescribed medications at home?

¿Tiene historial de?:

Do you have a history of:

Ingestión accidental			Accidental ingestions
Artritis			Arthritis
Asma			Asthma
Fibrilación auricular			Atrial fibrillation
Trastorno de coagulación de la sangre			Blood clotting disorder
Bronquitis			Bronchitis
Cáncer			Cancer
Parálisis cerebral			Cerebral palsy
Varicela			Chicken pox
Insuficiencia renal crónica			Chronic renal failure

PAST MEDICAL HISTORY

Complicaciones de la circuncisión	✓	✗	Circumcision complications
Labio y paladar leporino	✓	✗	Cleft lip/palate
Insuficiencia cardíaca congestiva (ICC)	✓	✗	Congestive heart failure (CHF)
Cortes, heridas, contusiones o heridas que no se han curado	✓	✗	Cuts, wounds, abrasions, or sores that have not healed
Problemas dentales	✓	✗	Dental problems
Condiciones dermatológicas	✓	✗	Dermatological conditions
Diabetes Mellitus Tipo 1 (insulinodependiente)	✓	✗	Diabetes mellitus Type 1 (IDDM)
Diabetes Mellitus Tipo 2	✓	✗	Diabetes mellitus Type 2
Enfisema	✓	✗	Emphysema
Disfunción del sistema endocrino	✓	✗	Endocrine system dysfunction
Epiglotitis	✓	✗	Epiglottitis
Reflujo gastroesofágico	✓	✗	Gastric esophageal reflux disease (GERD)
Problemas genitales (hombres)	✓	✗	Genital problems (Male)
Problemas ginecológicos	✓	✗	Gynecological problems
VIH/SIDA	✓	✗	HIV/AIDs
Problemas de la audición	✓	✗	Hearing problems

PAST MEDICAL HISTORY

22

Español			English
Infarto	✓	✗	*Heart attack*
Hemofilia	✓	✗	*Hemophilia*
Hepatitis A	✓	✗	*Hepatitis A*
Hepatitis B	✓	✗	*Hepatitis B*
Hepatitis C	✓	✗	*Hepatitis C*
Alta presión	✓	✗	*High blood pressure*
Problemas del sistema inmunológico	✓	✗	*Immune system conditions*
Problemas intestinales	✓	✗	*Intestinal conditions*
Meningitis	✓	✗	*Meningitis*
Mononucleosis	✓	✗	*Mononucleosis*
Enterocolitis necrotizante	✓	✗	*Necrotizing enterocolitis*
Trasplante de órganos	✓	✗	*Organ transplant*
Agresión física o sexual	✓	✗	*Physical/ sexual assault*
Neumonía	✓	✗	*Pneumonia*
Problemas psiquiátricos	✓	✗	*Psychiatric conditions*
Fisioterapia para una lesión	✓	✗	*Physical therapy for an injury*

PAST MEDICAL HISTORY

Embolia pulmonar	✓	✗	Pulmonary embolism
Cirugía reciente	✓	✗	Recent surgery
Dermatofitosis / pie de atleta	✓	✗	Ringworm/ athlete's foot
El VSR/Bronquiolitis	✓	✗	RSV/Bronchiolitis
Escabiosis	✓	✗	Scabies
Escoliosis	✓	✗	Scoliosis
Convulsiones o problemas neurológicos	✓	✗	Seizures or neurological conditions
Convulsiones febriles	✓	✗	Febrile seizures
Crisis drepanocítica	✓	✗	Sickle cell crises
Espina bífida	✓	✗	Spina bifida
Taquicardia supraventricular (SVT)	✓	✗	Supra ventricular tachycardia (SVT)
Candidiasis bucal / infecciones causadas por levaduras candidas	✓	✗	Thrush/ yeast infections
Fístulas transesofágicas	✓	✗	Transesophageal fistulas
Úlceras o problemas estomacales	✓	✗	Ulcers or stomach conditions
Problemas de la vista	✓	✗	Vision problems

INITIAL PROCEDURAL

24

BLOOD PRESSURE

Le voy a tomar la presión arterial. Tal vez sienta incomodidad en el brazo pero solo por un momento.

I am going to take your blood pressure. Your arm may be briefly uncomfortable but only for a moment.

BLOOD SAMPLE

Tengo que utilizar una jeringa para obtener una muestra de sangre. Tal vez le arda brevemente pero esto es importante hacerlo para nosotros entender mejor cómo ayudarlo.

I need to use a needle to get a blood sample. This may sting briefly, but is important so we can better understand how to help you.

CATHETER

Tengo que colocarle un tubo en la vejiga. Esto va a ser incómodo momentáneamente.

I need to put a tube in your bladder. This will be uncomfortable for a moment.

EKG

Voy a colocarle unos adhesivos en los brazos y/o el tórax para medir la actividad eléctrica del corazón. Por favor no se mueva. Esto no le va a doler.

I am going to put some stickers on your arms and/or chest to measure the electrical activity of your heart. Please stay very still. This will not hurt.

IV

Voy a colocarle suero. Va a sentir una punzada brevemente pero esto es importante hacerlo para poder administrarle medicamentos.

I am going to start an IV. This may sting briefly, but is important so we can give you medication.

RESPIRATORY

Tengo que escuchar los pulmones. Por favor, respire normalmente.

I need to listen to your lungs. Please breathe normally.

TEMPERATURE

Le voy a tomar la temperatura con un termómetro. Por favor, abra la boca.

I am going to take your temperature with a thermometer. Please open your mouth.

URINE SAMPLE

Por favor, orine en este vaso. Cuando haya terminado, por favor tápelo y entrégueme la muestra.

Please urinate in this cup. When you are finished please secure the lid on top and give the sample to me.

CARDIOLOGY

26

Hola, soy un(a) profesional de la salud. No hablo español.

Hello, I am a healthcare professional. I do not speak Spanish.

Respóndame solo sí o no .

Only respond to me "yes" or "no."

ACUTE CARDIAC HISTORY

¿Siente dolor en el pecho?

Do you have chest pain?

Por favor, señale (en este dibujo de una persona) donde tiene dolor.

Please point (on this picture of a person) to where you have pain.

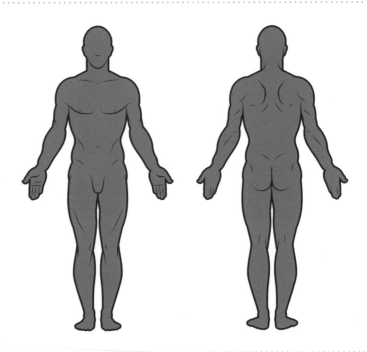

¿Cuándo comenzó el dolor?
When did your pain begin?

MINUTOS   10   20   30   40   50   60
MINUTES

HORAS   2   4   6   8   10   12   14   16   18   20   22
HOURS

DÍAS   1   2   3   4   5   6   7   8   9   10   >
DAYS

¿Qué estaba haciendo cuando empezó el dolor?
What were you doing when the pain began?

✓ Estaba parado
   Standing

✓ Durmiendo
   Sleeping

✓ Sentado
   Sitting

✓ Comiendo
   Eating

✓ Corriendo
   Running

✓ Fumando
   Smoking

✓ Caminando
   Walking

✓ Actividad sexual
   Sexual activity

✓ Montando bicicleta
   Riding bicycle

✓ Manejando un automóvil
   Driving car

✓ Levantando objetos pesados
   Lifting heavy objects

✓ Nadando
   Swimming

¿El dolor de pecho empeora con el ejercicio / actividad?
Does the chest pain get worse with exertion/activity?

¿Ha tenido una lesión en el pecho recientemente?
Have you recently had a physical injury to your chest?

¿Le duele cuando presiono el pecho hacia abajo?
Does it hurt when I press down on your chest?

¿Le duele cuando respira?
Does it hurt when you breathe in?

¿El dolor del pecho lo hace sentir que le falta el aire?
Does your chest pain make you short of breath?

¿El dolor del pecho lo hace sentir náuseas?
Does your chest pain make you feel nauseated?

¿El dolor del pecho lo hace vomitar?
Does your chest pain make you vomit?

¿Siente un sudor frío cuando comienza
el dolor en el pecho?
Do you have a cold sweat when your chest pain begins?

¿Se pone pálido cuando le empieza el dolor?
Do you get pale when your chest pain begins?

¿Ha tenido un ataque al corazón en el pasado?
Have you had a heart attack?

¿Le duele el pecho como la última vez que
tuvo un ataque al corazón?
Does your chest pain feel like the last time you had a heart attack?

¿Cómo describiría el dolor?
How would you describe your chest pain?

✔ **Que duele** Aching	✔ **Que desgarra** Ripping
✔ **Abrazador** Burning	✔ **Que irradia** Radiating
✔ **Con espasmos** Cramping	✔ **Agudo** Sharp
✔ **Devastador** Crushing	✔ **Fulgurante** Shooting
✔ **Que incomoda** Discomfort	✔ **Que resiente** Sore
✔ **Sordo** Dull	✔ **Que causa espasmos** Spasms
✔ **Que produce pesadez** Heaviness	✔ **Que aprieta** Squeezing
✔ **Que produce picazón** Itching	✔ **Lacerante** Stabbing
✔ **En oleadas punzantes** Jabbing	✔ **Que desgarra** Tearing
✔ **Persistente** Nagging	✔ **Sensible** Tender
✔ **Que acalambra** Numbness	✔ **Palpitante** Throbbing
✔ **Penetrante** Penetrating	✔ **Que oprime** Tightness
✔ **Con palpitaciones** Pounding	✔ **Que cansa** Tiring
✔ **Que ocasiona presión** Pressure	✔ **No puedo describirlo.** I can't describe it.

¿El dolor irradia o se traslada a otra área de su cuerpo?

Does the pain radiate or move to another area of your body?

Si el dolor se irradia, por favor señale sobre su propio cuerpo donde se traslada.

If the pain radiates, please point on your own body where it goes.

Por favor, indique (en la siguiente escala) la intensidad de su dolor.

Please point (on this scale) to rate your pain.

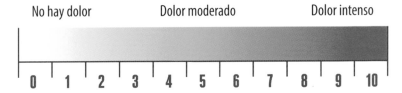

¿El dolor es constante o intermitente?

Is the pain constant or does it come and go?

 Constante
Constant

 Intermitente
Comes and goes

¿Ha tomado usted nitroglicerina hoy?

Have you taken nitroglycerin today?

¿La nitroglicerina le disminuye el dolor en el pecho?

Did the nitroglycerin improve your chest pain?

¿Ha tomado aspirina hoy?
Have you taken any aspirin today?

¿Ha tomado Viagra, Levitra o Cialis
(medicamentos para la disfunción eréctil) durante las
últimas 24 horas?
Have you taken Viagra, Levitra, or Cialis
(medications for erectile dysfunction) within the last 24 hours?

¿Con cuántas almohadas duerme en la noche?
How many pillows do you sleep on at night?

0   1   2   3   4   5   >

¿Ese es el número de almohadas normal para usted?
Is this number of pillows normal for you?

¿Usted se despierta en la noche y tiene que sentarse
o abrir la ventana para recuperar el aire?
Do you wake up at night and have to sit up or
open the window to catch your breath?

¿Tiene tos?
Do you have a cough?

¿Tiene hinchazón en las piernas?
Do you have leg swelling?

¿Esta hinchazón en las piernas es algo nuevo?
Is this leg swelling new?

CARDIOLOGY

32

CARDIAC PROCEDURAL

Le voy a dar algo de oxígeno mediante el uso de una máscara que va en la cara o dentro la nariz. Puede ser incómodo.

I am going to give you some oxygen either by a mask that goes over you face or up your nose. It may be uncomfortable.

¿El oxígeno le está ayudando con el dolor en el pecho y/o la dificultad para respirar?

Is the oxygen helping your chest pain and/or shortness of breath?

Aquí tiene aspirina masticable. Por favor, mastíquela y tráguesela.

Here is some chewable aspirin. Please chew it up and swallow.

Le voy a administrar nitroglicerina. Por favor abra la boca y coloque la lengua en el paladar. Le voy a rociar el medicamento debajo de la lengua o le voy a colocar una pequeña tableta debajo de la lengua. Esto podría ocasionarle dolor de cabeza.

I am going to give you some nitroglycerin. Please open your mouth and put your tongue to the roof of your mouth. I will either spray some medicine under your tongue or place a small medicine tablet under your tongue. This may give you a headache.

Voy a colocarle unos adhesivos en los brazos y/o el tórax para medir la actividad eléctrica del corazón. Por favor, no se mueva. Esto no le va a doler.

I am going to put some stickers on your arms and/or chest to measure the electrical activity of your heart. Please stay very still. This will not hurt.

Voy a colocarle suero. Va a sentir una punzada brevemente pero esto es importante hacerlo para poder administrarle medicamentos.

I am going to start an IV. This may sting briefly, but is important so we can give you medication.

Tengo que utilizar una jeringa para obtener una muestra de sangre. Tal vez le arda brevemente pero esto es importante hacerlo para nosotros entender mejor cómo ayudarlo.

I need to use a needle to get a blood sample. This may sting briefly, but is important so we can better understand how to help you.

Le voy a administrar medicamento en el suero.

I am going to give you medication through your IV.

¿Cómo describiría en este momento el dolor en el pecho?

How would you now describe your chest pain?

 Mejor
Better

 Lo mismo
Same

 Peor
Worse

 Se me quitó
Gone

¿Ha cambiado de característica el dolor que siente en el pecho?

Has the quality of your chest pain changed?

CARDIOLOGY

34

PAST CARDIAC HISTORY

¿Usted tiene la presión sanguínea alta?
Do you have high blood pressure?

¿Tiene diabetes?
Do you have diabetes?

¿Ha tenido un infarto?
Have you had a heart attack?

¿Cuántos infartos ha tenido?
How many heart attacks have you had?

0   1   2   3   4   5   >

¿Le han colocado stents (prótesis endovascular)?
Have you had stents placed?

¿Alguna vez ha tomado medicamentos
destructores de coágulos?
Have you ever received clot-busting drugs?

¿Ha tenido una embolia pulmonar?
Have you had a pulmonary embolism?

¿Ha tenido una trombosis venosa profunda?
Have you had a deep vein thrombosis?

¿Usted toma aspirina diariamente?
Do you take aspirin on a daily basis?

¿Usa usted diluyentes de la sangre?
Are you on blood thinners?

¿Le han realizado una cirugía de derivación coronaria?
Have you had a heart bypass surgery?

¿Usted sufre de vasos sanguíneos en mal estado?
Do you have bad blood vessels?

¿Ha tenido un aneurisma?
Have you had an aneurysm?

¿Tiene implantado un marcapasos o desfibrilador?
Do you have an implanted pacemaker/defibrillator?

¿Tiene historial de fibrilación auricular?
Do you have a history of atrial fibrillation?

¿Tiene historial de edema pulmonar?
Do you have a history of pulmonary edema?

¿Tiene historial de enfermedad pulmonar obstructiva crónica?
Do you have a history of chronic obstructive pulmonary disease (COPD)?

¿Tiene historial de enfisema?
Do you have a history of emphysema?

¿Tiene historial de bronquitis?
Do you have a history of bronchitis?

ENDOCRINOLOGY

36

ACUTE ENDOCRINE HISTORY

¿Tiene diabetes?
Do you have diabetes?

¿Cuándo fue la última vez que se revisó el nivel de azúcar en la sangre?
When was the last time you checked your blood sugar level?

DÍAS										
DAYS	1	2	3	4	5	6	7 >			

SEMANAS										
WEEKS	1	2	3	4	5	6	7	8	9	10 >

MESES										
MONTHS	1	2	3	4	5	6	7	8	9	10 >

AÑOS										
YEARS	1	2	3	4	5	6	7	8	9	10 >

¿Cuál era su nivel de azúcar en la sangre la última vez que se la revisó?
What was your blood sugar level when you checked it last?

Bajo   Alto

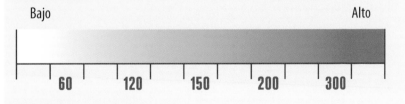

60   120   150   200   300

¿Se aplica insulina?
Do you take insulin?

 Sí
Yes

 No
No

 Ya no me aplico.
Not any more.

¿Cuándo se aplica normalmente la insulina?

When do you normally take your insulin?

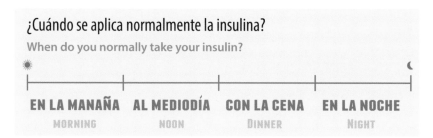

EN LA MANAÑA	AL MEDIODÍA	CON LA CENA	EN LA NOCHE
MORNING	NOON	DINNER	NIGHT

¿Cuándo fue la última vez que se aplicó insulina?

When was the last time you took your insulin?

DÍAS DAYS	1	2	3	4	5	6	7	>

SEMANAS WEEKS	1	2	3	4	5	6	7	8	9	10	>

MESES MONTHS	1	2	3	4	5	6	7	8	9	10	>

ENDOCRINE PROCEDURAL

Le voy a revisar el nivel de azúcar en la sangre. Va a sentir un pinchazo brevemente.

I am going to check your blood sugar. This might sting briefly.

Le voy a hacer una prueba de tolerancia a la glucosa. Va a sentir un pinchazo brevemente. Después que se tome el líquido revisaremos periódicamente sus niveles de azúcar en la sangre.

I am going to give you glucose tolerance test. This may sting briefly.
After drinking this liquid we will test your blood sugar levels periodically.

ENDOCRINOLOGY

38

Por favor, coma para que aumenten los niveles de azúcar en sangre.
Please eat so we can increase your blood sugar levels.

Le voy a administrar glucagon.
I am going to give you some glucagon.

Le voy a administrar insulina.
I am going to give you some insulin.

PAST ENDOCRINE HISTORY

¿Tiene diabetes tipo 1 o tipo 2?
Do you have Type 1 or Type 2 Diabetes?

¿Su nivel de azúcar en la sangre normalmente pasa de más de 120 [mg/dl]?
Does your blood sugar level typically run over 120 [mg/dl]?

¿Su nivel de azúcar en la sangre normalmente pasa de menos de 60 [mg/dl]?
Does your blood sugar level typically run under 60 [mg/dl]?

¿Usted toma medicamentos para la diabetes vía oral?
Do you take oral medication for your diabetes?

¿Alguna vez ha sido hospitalizado por tener niveles muy altos de azúcar en la sangre?
Have you ever been hospitalized for having very high blood sugar levels?

¿Alguna vez ha sido hospitalizado por tener niveles muy bajos de azúcar en la sangre?
Have you ever been hospitalized for having very low blood sugar levels?

Hola, soy un(a) profesional de la salud. No hablo español.
Hello, I am a healthcare professional. I do not speak Spanish.

Respóndame solo sí o no .
Only respond to me "yes" or "no."

ACUTE GASTROINTESTINAL HISTORY

¿Tiene dolor en la boca?
Do you have pain in your mouth?

¿Siente dolor al tragar?
Do you have pain when you swallow?

¿Tiene alguna lesión en la boca?
Do you have any lesions in your mouth?

¿Siente acidez estomacal sin haber comido alimentos?
Do you have heartburn without food?

¿Siente acidez estomacal sin haber comido?
Do you have heartburn without eating?

¿Siente náuseas?
Are you nauseated?

¿Cuántas veces siente náuseas durante el día?
How often are you nauseated during a day?

Rara vez	A veces	A menudo	Siempre

GASTROINTESTINAL

¿Siente náuseas antes o después de comer?
Does the nausea come before or after eating?

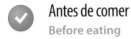

✓ **Antes de comer**
Before eating

✓ **Después de comer**
After eating

✓ **Ambos**
Both

✓ **En ninguno de los casos**
Neither

✓ **No lo sé.**
I don't know.

¿Usted vomita con regularidad?
Do you vomit regularly?

¿Cuánto a menudo vomita?
How often do you vomit?

HORAS   2   4   6   8   10   12   14   16   18   20   22   >
HOURS

¿De qué color es el vómito?
What color is the vomit?

✓ **Negro**
Black

✓ **Rojo intenso**
Bright red

✓ **Transparente**
Clear

✓ **Rojo oscuro**
Dark red

✓ **Verde**
Green

✓ **Mucoso**
Mucousy

✓ **Rojo**
Red

✓ **Marrón claro**
Tan

✓ **Alimento no digerido**
Undigested food

✓ **Amarillo**
Yellow

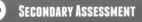
GASTROINTESTINAL

¿Hay sangre en el vómito?
Is there blood in the vomit?

¿Qué tanta cantidad de sangre hay en el vómito?
How much blood is in the vomit?

Ninguna	Un poco	La mitad	Mucho	Sólo sangre

¿Vomita antes o después de comer?
Does the vomit come before or after eating?

 Antes
Before

 En ninguno de los casos
Neither

 Después
After

 No lo sé.
I don't know.

 Ambos
Both

¿Puede usted tragar y retener los líquidos?
Can you swallow and and keep down liquids?

¿Puede usted tragar y retener los sólidos?
Can you swallow and keep down solids?

¿Siente dolor en el estómago?
Do you have abdominal pain?

Por favor, señale sobre su propio abdomen exactamente donde siente dolor.
Please point on your own abdomen exactly where you have abdominal pain.

¿Cuándo comenzó el dolor?

When did your pain begin?

MINUTOS MINUTES	10	20	30	40	50	60					
HORAS HOURS	2	4	6	8	10	12	14	16	18	20	22
DÍAS DAYS	1	2	3	4	5	6	7	8	9	10	>
SEMANAS WEEKS	1	2	3	4	5	6	7	8	9	10	>
MESES MONTHS	1	2	3	4	5	6	7	8	9	10	>
AÑOS YEARS	1	2	3	4	5	6	7	8	9	10	>

¿Cómo describiría el inicio del dolor?

How would you describe the onset of your pain?

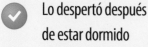 Lo despertó después de estar dormido
Awakened from sleep

Gradual
Gradual

Continuo
Ongoing

 Progresivo
Progressive

 Repentino
Sudden

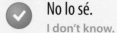 No lo sé.
I don't know.

¿El dolor empeora al comer?
Does the pain get worse with eating?

¿El dolor disminuye al comer?
Does the pain get better with eating?

¿El dolor empeora al moverse?
Does the pain get worse when moving?

¿El dolor empeora al quedarse quieto?
Does the pain get worse when staying still?

¿Qué hace que el dolor disminuya?
What makes the pain better?

 Al moverse
Moving

 El hielo/el frío
Ice/cold

 Al posicionarse
Adjusting your position

 El calor
Heat

 Medicamentos
Medication

 La actividad
Physical activity

¿Qué hace que el dolor empeore?
What makes the pain worse?

 Al estar parado
Standing

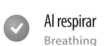 **Al respirar**
Breathing

 Al tocarse o que lo toquen
Touch

 Al comer
Eating

 Al orinar
Urination

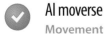 **Al moverse**
Movement

 Al caminar
Walking

GASTROINTESTINAL

44

¿Cómo describiría el dolor?
How would you describe your pain?

✔ Que duele — Aching	✔ Que desgarra — Ripping
✔ Abrazador — Burning	✔ Que irradia — Radiating
✔ Con espasmos — Cramping	✔ Agudo — Sharp
✔ Devastador — Crushing	✔ Fulgurante — Shooting
✔ Que incomoda — Discomfort	✔ Que resiente — Sore
✔ Sordo — Dull	✔ Que causa espasmos — Spasms
✔ Que produce pesadez — Heaviness	✔ Que aprieta — Squeezing
✔ Que produce picazón — Itching	✔ Lacerante — Stabbing
✔ En oleadas punzantes — Jabbing	✔ Que desgarra — Tearing
✔ Persistente — Nagging	✔ Sensible — Tender
✔ Que acalambra — Numbness	✔ Palpitante — Throbbing
✔ Penetrante — Penetrating	✔ Que oprime — Tightness
✔ Con palpitaciones — Pounding	✔ Que cansa — Tiring
✔ Que ocasiona presión — Pressure	✔ No puedo describirlo. — I can't describe it.

¿El dolor irradia o se traslada a otra área de su cuerpo?
Does the pain radiate or move to another area of your body?

Si el dolor se irradia, por favor señale sobre su propio cuerpo donde se traslada.
If the pain radiates, please point on your own body where it goes.

Por favor, indique (en la siguiente escala) la intensidad de su dolor.
Please point (on this scale) to rate your pain.

No hay dolor   Dolor moderado   Dolor intenso

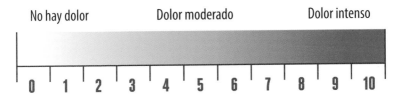

¿El dolor es constante o intermitente?
Is the pain constant or does it come and go?

 Constante
Constant

 Intermitente
Comes and goes

¿Cuándo fue la última vez que defecó?
When was your last bowel movement?

| **DÍAS** | 1 | 2 | 3 | 4 | 5 | 6 | 7 | 8 | 9 | 10 | > |
| DAYS | | | | | | | | | | | |

| **SEMANAS** | 1 | 2 | 3 | 4 | 5 | 6 | 7 | 8 | 9 | 10 | > |
| WEEKS | | | | | | | | | | | |

¿Ha perdido el control de los intestinos (incontinencia)?
Have you lost control of your bowels (incontinence)?

¿Tiene deposiciones normales?
Do you have normal bowel movements?

¿Cómo describiría su más reciente deposición?
How would you describe your most recent bowel movement?

✓	**Negra** Black	✓	**Roja** Red
✓	**Marrón** Brown	✓	**Con vetas rojas** Red streaks
✓	**Arcilla** Clay	✓	**Marrón clara** Tan
✓	**Verde** Green	✓	**Amarilla** Yellow
✓	**Meconio** Meconium	✓	**Blanca** White

¿De qué tamaño describiría su más reciente deposición?
How large was your most recent bowel movement?

Pequeña   Mediana   Grande

├─────────────────────┼─────────────────────┤

¿De dónde procede la más reciente deposición?
Where did your most recent bowel movement come from?

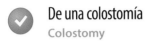 **De una colostomía**
Colostomy

 De un sistema de manejo fecal
Fecal management system

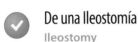 **De una Ileostomía**
Ileostomy

 Del recto
Rectum

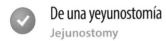 **De una yeyunostomía**
Jejunostomy

¿Había sangre presente en la materia fecal?
Did your stool have blood in it?

¿Tiene diarrea?
Do you have diarrhea?

¿Tiene estreñimiento?
Are you constipated?

¿Cuándo fue la última vez que hizo una deposición normal?
When was the last time you had a normal bowel movement?

DÍAS   1   2   3   4   5   6   7   8   9   10   >
DAYS

SEMANAS   1   2   3   4   5   6   7   8   9   10   >
WEEKS

¿Con qué frecuencia hace deposiciones?
How often are you moving your bowels?

1   2   3   4   5   6   7   >   **CADA DÍA**

¿Cómo describiría las heces fecales?
How would you describe your stool?

✓ **Normales**
Normal

✓ **Anormales**
Abnormal

✓ **Suaves**
Soft

✓ **Dolorosas**
Painful

✓ **Líquidas**
Liquid

¿Siente ganas de defecar pero no puede?
Do you feel the urge to move your bowels but can't?

✓ ✗

¿Tiene picazón?
Do you have itching?

✓ ✗

¿Ha notado erupciones cutáneas en sus glúteos y recto?
Have you noticed rashes around your buttocks/rectum?

✓ ✗

¿Qué medicamentos usa usted para cualquiera de estos problemas?
What medications have you taken for any of these problems?

✓ **Crema tópica**
Topical cream

✓ **Otros**
Other

✓ **Ungüento**
Ointment

✓ **Nada**
Nothing

✓ **Medicamento vía oral**
Oral medication

¿Los medicamentos le aliviaron el malestar?
Did the medications alleviate your discomfort?

? ✓ ✗

GASTROINTESTINAL PROCEDURAL

Voy a presionar en varios lugares del abdomen para examinarlo.
Esto puede doler y/o ser incómodo.

I am going to press down in various places on your abdomen to examine it.
This may hurt and/or be uncomfortable.

Le voy a administrar medicamento para ablandar las heces fecales.

I am going to give you some medication to soften your stool.

Le voy a administrar líquidos en el suero.

I am going to give you fluids through your IV.

PAST GASTROINTESTINAL HISTORY

¿Ha tenido alguna cirugía abdominal?

Have you had abdominal surgery?

¿Usted padece de enfermedad de Crohn?

Do you have Crohn's Disease?

¿Tiene síndrome de intestino irritable?

Do you have Irritable Bowel Syndrome?

¿Alguna vez ha tenido una hernia?

Have you ever had a hernia?

¿Le han sacado?:	La vesícula	✓	✗	Gall Bladder
Have you had this removed:	El bazo	✓	✗	Spleen
	El apéndice	✓	✗	Appendix

GASTROINTESTINAL

50

¿Tiene historial de?:

Do you have a history of:

Colecistitis	✓	✗	*Cholecystitis*
Sangrado intestinal	✓	✗	*Intestinal bleeding*
Problemas de vesícula	✓	✗	*Gall bladder problems*
Cálculos biliares	✓	✗	*Gall stones*
Problemas de hígado	✓	✗	*Liver problems*
Hepatitis A	✓	✗	*Hepatitis A*
Hepatitis B	✓	✗	*Hepatitis B*
Hepatitis C	✓	✗	*Hepatitis C*
Cirrosis del hígado	✓	✗	*Cirrhosis of the liver*
Pancreatitis	✓	✗	*Pancreatitis*
Problemas del bazo	✓	✗	*Spleen problems*
Problemas de colitis ulcerosa	✓	✗	*Ulcerative colitis*
Problemas de obstrucción intestinal	✓	✗	*Bowel obstructions*
Sangrado en el intestino delgado	✓	✗	*Bleeding in small intestine*
Sangrado en el intestino grueso	✓	✗	*Bleeding in large intestine (colon)*
Problemas de riñones	✓	✗	*Kidney problems*

ACUTE GYNECOLOGICAL HISTORY

¿Tiene dolor en la pelvis?
Do you have pain in your pelvis?

Por favor, indique (en la siguiente escala) la intensidad de su dolor.
Please point (on this scale) to rate your pain.

No hay dolor   Dolor moderado   Dolor intenso

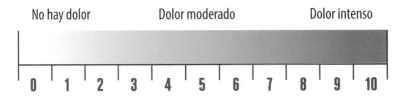

0   1   2   3   4   5   6   7   8   9   10

¿Cuándo comenzó el dolor?
When did your pain begin?

MINUTOS MINUTES	10	20	30	40	50	60					
HORAS HOURS	2	4	6	8	10	12	14	16	18	20	22
DÍAS DAYS	1	2	3	4	5	6	7	8	9	10	>
SEMANAS WEEKS	1	2	3	4	5	6	7	8	9	10	>
MESES MONTHS	1	2	3	4	5	6	7	8	9	10	>

¿Cómo describiría el inicio del dolor?
How would you describe the onset of your pain?

✓ **Lo despertó después de estar dormido**
Awakened from sleep

✓ **Gradual**
Gradual

✓ **Continuo**
Ongoing

✓ **Progresivo**
Progressive

✓ **Repentino**
Sudden

✓ **No lo sé.**
I don't know.

¿Qué hace que el dolor empeore?
What makes the pain worse?

✓ **Al respirar**
Breathing

✓ **Al comer**
Eating

✓ **Al moverse**
Movement

✓ **Al estar parado**
Standing

✓ **Al estar acostado**
Lying down

✓ **Al defecar**
Defecating

✓ **Al tocarse o que lo toquen**
Touch

✓ **Al orinar**
Urination

✓ **Al caminar**
Walking

✓ **Al toser**
Coughing

✓ **Al correr**
Running

✓ **Actividad sexual**
Sexual activity

¿Cómo describiría el dolor?
How would you describe your pain?

✓ Que duele
Aching

✓ Abrazador
Burning

✓ Con espasmos
Cramping

✓ Devastador
Crushing

✓ Que incomoda
Discomfort

✓ Sordo
Dull

✓ Que produce pesadez
Heaviness

✓ Que produce picazón
Itching

✓ En oleadas punzantes
Jabbing

✓ Persistente
Nagging

✓ Que acalambra
Numbness

✓ Penetrante
Penetrating

✓ Con palpitaciones
Pounding

✓ Que ocasiona presión
Pressure

✓ Que desgarra
Ripping

✓ Que irradia
Radiating

✓ Agudo
Sharp

✓ Fulgurante
Shooting

✓ Que resiente
Sore

✓ Que causa espasmos
Spasms

✓ Que aprieta
Squeezing

✓ Lacerante
Stabbing

✓ Que desgarra
Tearing

✓ Sensible
Tender

✓ Palpitante
Throbbing

✓ Que oprime
Tightness

✓ Que cansa
Tiring

✓ No puedo describirlo.
I can't describe it.

¿El dolor irradia o se traslada a otra área de su cuerpo?

Does the pain radiate or move to another area of your body?

Si el dolor se irradia, por favor señale sobre su propio cuerpo donde se traslada.

If the pain radiates, please point on your own body where it goes.

Por favor, indique (en la siguiente escala) la intensidad de su dolor.

Please point (on this scale) to rate your pain.

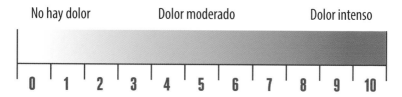

¿El dolor es constante o intermitente?

Is the pain constant or does it come and go?

 Constante
Constant

 Intermitente
Comes and goes

¿Tiene sangrado vaginal anormal?

Do you have abnormal vaginal bleeding?

¿Este sangrado ocurre durante su período normal o no ocurre durante su período?

Does this bleeding occur during your normal period or not during your period?

¿Cuántas toallas sanitarias ha usado desde que comenzó a sangrar?
How many pads have you gone through since your bleeding started?

0   1   2   3   4   5

¿El sangrado es doloroso?
Is the bleeding painful?

¿Tiene secreción vaginal anormal?
Do you have an abnormal vaginal discharge?

¿De qué color es?
What color is it?

 Negra
Black

 Roja
Red

 Marrón
Brown

 Amarilla
Yellow

 Verde
Green

¿Tiene mal olor la secreción vaginal?
Does the abnormal vaginal discharge smell bad?

¿Cómo describiría la secreción vaginal anormal?
How would you describe the abnormal vaginal discharge?

 Líquida
Liquid

 Pegajosa
Sticky

 Mucosa
Mucus-like

 Sólida
Solid

GYNECOLOGY

56

GYNECOLOGY PROCEDURAL

Por favor, cámbiese de ropa y póngase esta bata.

Please change out of your clothes and into this gown.

Por favor, acuéstese en la mesa y ponga los pies en los estribos.

Please lie down on the table and put your feet into the stirrups.

Voy a colocarle este espéculo en la vagina para examinarla.

Primero va a sentir que la toco y después va a sentir el espéculo.

Esto puede ser un poco incómodo.

I am going to place this speculum into your vagina to examine it.

First you will feel my touch, then you will feel the speculum.

This may be uncomfortable.

Voy a recoger una muestra del interior de la vagina.

Esto puede ser un poco incómodo.

I am going to swab the inside of your vagina and take a sample.

This may be uncomfortable.

Por favor, relájese.

Please relax.

Hemos terminado.

We are done.

Por favor, póngase su ropa.

Please change back into your own clothes.

PAST GYNECOLOGICAL HISTORY

¿Ya empezó su ciclo menstrual?
Have you started your menstrual cycle yet?

¿Su período/ciclo menstrual es regular?
Is your period/menstrual cycle regular?

Indique cuántas semanas han pasado desde la última menstruación.
Indicate how many weeks have passed since your last menstrual period.

| **SEMANAS** WEEKS | 1 | 2 | 3 | 4 | 5 | 6 | 7 | 8 | 9 | 10 | > |

| **MESES** MONTHS | 1 | 2 | 3 | 4 | 5 | 6 | 7 | 8 | 9 | 10 | > |

| **AÑOS** YEARS | 1 | 2 | 3 | 4 | 5 | 6 | 7 | 8 | 9 | 10 | > |

¿Qué edad tenía cuando tuvo su primer período?
How old were you when you had your first period?

10   11   12   13   14   15   16   17   18   >

¿Cuánto le dura el período normal?
How long does your normal period last?

| **DÍAS** DAYS | 1 | 2 | 3 | 4 | 5 | 6 | 7 | 8 | 9 | 10 | > |

¿Cómo describiría normalmente el color de la sangre del período?

How would you normally describe the color of your period blood?

| Rojo claro | Rojo | Oscuro |

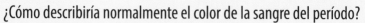

¿Cuántas toallas sanitarias o tampones usa normalmente durante su período?

How many pads, sanitary napkins, or tampons do you normally go through during your period?

0   1   2   3   4   5   6   7   8   9   10   >

¿Normalmente tiene cólicos durante su período?

Do you normally have cramps during your period?

?

Por favor, indique (en la siguiente escala) la intensidad de su dolor.

Please point (on this scale) to rate your pain.

| No hay dolor | Dolor moderado | Dolor intenso |

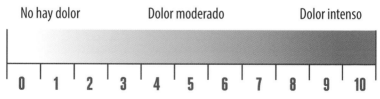

0   1   2   3   4   5   6   7   8   9   10

¿Ha estado embarazada alguna vez?
Have you ever been pregnant?

Indique el número de veces que ha estado embarazada.
Indicate how many times you have been pregnant.

1 2 3 4 5 6 7 8 9 10 >

¿Tiene hijos?
Do you have any children?

Indique el número de hijos que tiene.
Indicate how many children you have.

1 2 3 4 5 6 7 8 9 10 >

¿Alguna vez le han practicado un aborto o ha tenido un aborto espontaneo?
Have you ever had an abortion or a miscarriage?

Indique el número de abortos provocados o abortos espontáneos que haya tenido.
Indicate how many abortions or miscarriages you have had.

1 2 3 4 5 6 7 8 9 10 >

¿Alguna vez ha tenido un embarazo ectópico anterior?
Have you ever had a previous ectopic pregnancy?

¿Ha tenido complicaciones con un embarazo anterior?
Have you had complications with a past pregnancy?

¿Cómo describiría su actividad sexual?
How would best describe your sexual activity?

 Inactiva
Inactive

 Activa
Active

No muy activa
Not very active

Frecuente
Frequent

 Moderada
Moderate

¿Cuántos compañeros sexuales ha tenido?
How many sexual partners have you had?

1   2   3   4   5   6   7   8   9   10   >

¿Tiene relaciones sexuales con hombres, mujeres, o con ambos?
Do you have sex with men, women, or both?

 Hombre
Male

 Mujer
Female

 Ambos
Both

¿Usa anticonceptivos?
Do you use contraception?

 Sí
Yes

 No
No

 Sí, a veces
Sometimes

¿Alguna vez ha tenido relaciones sexuales sin protección?
Have you ever had unprotected sex?

¿Cuándo fue la última vez que tuvo relaciones sexuales sin protección?

When was the last time you had unprotected sex?

HORAS HOURS	2	4	6	8	10	12	14	16	18	20	22
DÍAS DAYS	1	2	3	4	5	6	7	8	9	10	>
SEMANAS WEEKS	1	2	3	4	5	6	7	8	9	10	>
MESES MONTHS	1	2	3	4	5	6	7	8	9	10	>

¿Alguna vez ha contraído una enfermedad de transmisión sexual?

Have you ever contracted a sexually transmitted diseased?

¿Alguna vez ha sido víctima de violencia?

Have you ever been a victim of violence?

¿Ha sido víctima de violencia en los últimos 6 meses?

Have you been a victim of violence within the past 6 months?

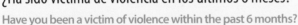

¿Alguien la ha obligado a tener relaciones sexuales sin su consentimiento?

Has anyone ever forced you into sexual activity unwillingly?

¿Las relaciones sexuales sin su consentimiento ocurrieron en los últimos 6 meses?

Did the unwanted sexual activity occur within the past 6 months?

NEUROLOGY

62

ACUTE NEUROLOGICAL HISTORY

¿Los síntomas comenzaron hoy?

Did your symptoms begin today?

Si los síntomas empezaron hoy, por favor indique cuando empezaron.

If the symptoms began today please indicate when they began.

AM	1	2	3	4	5	6	7	8	9	10	11	12
PM	1	2	3	4	5	6	7	8	9	10	11	12

Si los síntomas empezaron antes del día de hoy, por favor indique cuando empezaron.

If the symptoms began before today please indicate when they began.

DÍAS Days	1	2	3	4	5	6	7	8	9	10	>
SEMANAS Weeks	1	2	3	4	5	6	7	8	9	10	>
MESES Months	1	2	3	4	5	6	7	8	9	10	>
AÑOS Years	1	2	3	4	5	6	7	8	9	10	>

FOR CAREGIVER/FAMILY/WITNESS

Por favor, indique cuándo aproximadamente se encontró al paciente.

Please indicate approximately when the patient was found.

AM	1	2	3	4	5	6	7	8	9	10	11	12
PM	1	2	3	4	5	6	7	8	9	10	11	12

¿Cuándo fue la última vez que al paciente se le vio normal?

When was the last time the patient seemed normal?

MINUTOS MINUTES	10	20	30	40	50	60					
HORAS HOURS	2	4	6	8	10	12	14	16	18	20	22
DÍAS DAYS	1	2	3	4	5	6	7	8	9	10	>
SEMANAS WEEKS	1	2	3	4	5	6	7	8	9	10	>
MESES MONTHS	1	2	3	4	5	6	7	8	9	10	>
AÑOS YEARS	1	2	3	4	5	6	7	8	9	10	>

BACK TO PATIENT

¿Tiene desmayos?
Are you having blackout spells?

¿Ha tenido desmayos en el pasado?
Have you had blackouts in the past?

¿Cuánto tiempo ha tenido desmayos?
How long have you had blackouts?

SEMANAS WEEKS	1	2	3	4	5	6	7	8	9	10	>
MESES MONTHS	1	2	3	4	5	6	7	8	9	10	>
AÑOS YEARS	1	2	3	4	5	6	7	8	9	10	>

¿Con qué frecuencia se desmaya?
How often do you have blackouts?

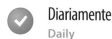 Diariamente
Daily

1-5 por mes
1-5 per month

 1-5 por semana
1-5 per week

1-5 por año
1-5 per year

¿Cuánto tiempo duran los desmayos?
How long do the blackouts last?

30 SEC | **1 MIN** | **5 MIN** | **15 MIN** | **30 MIN** | **1 HR** | **6 HR**

¿Puede anticipar cuando está a punto de desmayarse?
Can you tell when you are about to have a blackout?

¿Recuerda que se desmayó?
Do you remember having the blackout?

¿Los desmayos hacen que se contorsione o sacuda?
Do the blackouts cause you to twitch or jerk?

¿Los desmayos hacen que pierda el control de
la vejiga o los intestinos?
Do the blackouts cause you to lose control of your bladder or bowels?

¿Los desmayos hacen que se muerda la lengua o la mejilla?
Do the blackouts cause you to bite your tongue or cheek?

¿Después de los desmayos se siente confundido
o desorientado?
After the blackouts do you feel confused or disoriented?

¿Después de los desmayos se siente cansado?
After the blackouts do you feel tired?

¿Después de los desmayos se siente enojado o irritado?
After the blackouts do you feel angry or upset?

¿Es usted capaz de controlar los intestinos y/o la vejiga?
Are you able to control your bowels and/or bladder?

¿La pérdida de control de los intestinos y/o de la
vejiga ocurre de repente?
Did the loss of control of your bowels and/or bladder occur suddenly?

¿Ha tenido problemas de confusión o pérdida de la memoria?

Have you had any problems with confusion or loss of memory?

¿Cuándo comenzó la confusión o pérdida de la memoria?

When did the confusion or memory loss start?

MINUTOS MINUTES	10	20	30	40	50	60				
HORAS HOURS	2	4	6	8	10	12	14	16	18	20	22
DÍAS DAYS	1	2	3	4	5	6	7	8	9	10	>
SEMANAS WEEKS	1	2	3	4	5	6	7	8	9	10	>
MESES MONTHS	1	2	3	4	5	6	7	8	9	10	>
AÑOS YEARS	1	2	3	4	5	6	7	8	9	10	>

¿La confusión o pérdida de la memoria es constante o intermitente?

Is the confusion or memory loss constant or does it come and go?

 Constante
Constant

 Intermitente
Comes and goes

¿Tiene mareos o problemas de equilibrio?
Do you have dizziness or balance problems?

¿Ha tenido problemas de mareos o de equilibrio?
Have you had dizziness/balance problems in the past?

¿Tiene problemas de mareos o de equilibrio en la cabeza o en las piernas?
Do you have dizziness/balance problems in the head or in the legs?

 En la cabeza
Head

 Con ambos
Both

 En las piernas
Legs

 No
No

¿Cuándo comenzaron los problemas de mareo o de equilibrio?
When did the dizziness/balance problems start?

MINUTOS MINUTES	10	20	30	40	50	60				
HORAS HOURS	2	4	6	8	10	12	14	16	18	20	22
DÍAS DAYS	1	2	3	4	5	6	7	8	9	10	>
SEMANAS WEEKS	1	2	3	4	5	6	7	8	9	10	>
MESES MONTHS	1	2	3	4	5	6	7	8	9	10	>
AÑOS YEARS	1	2	3	4	5	6	7	8	9	10	>

¿Con qué frecuencia se siente mareado/desequilibrado?

How often do you feel dizzy/off balance?

 Diariamente
Daily

✓ **1-5 por semana**
1-5 per week

✓ **1-5 por mes**
1-5 per month

✓ **1-5 por año**
1-5 per year

¿Cuánto tiempo dura el mareo/problema de equilibrio?

How long does the dizziness/balance problem last?

30 SEC | **1 MIN** | **15 MIN** | **30 MIN** | **1 HR** | **6 HR** | **12 HR** >

¿Describiría sus mareos como una sensación en que todo da vueltas, aturdimiento o pérdida del equilibrio?

Would you describe your dizziness as a spinning, lightheaded, or off balance feeling?

 Mareos
Dizziness

 Aturdimiento
Lightheadedness

 Ambas cosas
Both

 No
No

¿El mareo empeora cuando se acuesta o se da vuelta?

Does the dizziness get worse when you lie down or roll over?

¿El mareo empeora cuando se para o camina?

Does the dizziness get worse when you stand up or walk?

¿Siente náuseas?

Do you feel nauseous?

¿Ha estado vomitando?
Have you been vomiting?

¿Ha estado sudando?
Have you been sweating?

¿Ha tenido pérdida de la audición últimamente?
Do you have recent hearing loss?

¿Siente dolor de oído?
Do you have ear pain?

¿Tiene palpitaciones?
Do you have palpitations?

¿Usted toma medicamentos para el mareo?
Do you take any medications for your dizziness?

¿Tiene dolor de cabeza?
Do you have a headache?

Por favor, señale en su propia cabeza donde siente los dolores de cabeza.
Please point to the location on your own head where the headaches are.

¿El dolor se traslada?
Does the pain move?

Por favor, señale en su propia cabeza hacia donde se desplaza el dolor.
Please point to the location on your own head where the pain moves.

¿Ha tenido dolores de cabeza en el pasado?
Have you had headaches in the past?

¿Este dolor de cabeza es diferente o igual a los anteriores dolores de cabeza?
Is this headache different or the same as your prior headaches?

 Igual
Same

 Diferente
Different

¿Cuándo comenzaron los dolores de cabeza?
When did the headaches start?

MINUTOS MINUTES	10	20	30	40	50	60					
HORAS HOURS	2	4	6	8	10	12	14	16	18	20	22
DÍAS DAYS	1	2	3	4	5	6	7	8	9	10	>
SEMANAS WEEKS	1	2	3	4	5	6	7	8	9	10	>
MESES MONTHS	1	2	3	4	5	6	7	8	9	10	>
AÑOS YEARS	1	2	3	4	5	6	7	8	9	10	>

¿Con qué frecuencia le dan dolores de cabeza?
How often do you get headaches?

 Nunca antes
Never before

 1-5 por mes
1-5 per month

Diariamente
Daily

1-5 por año
1-5 per year

 1-5 por semana
1-5 per week

¿Cuánto tiempo duran los dolores de cabeza?
How long do your headaches last?

30 SEC | **1 MIN** | **15 MIN** | **30 MIN** | **1 HR** | **6 HR** | **12 HR** >

¿Cómo describiría los dolores de cabeza?
How would you describe your headaches?

Palpitante
Throbbing

 Lacerante
Stabbing

Presión/dolor sordo
Pressure/dull

 Otro
Other

Por favor, indique (en la siguiente escala) la intensidad de su dolor.
Please point (on this scale) to rate your pain.

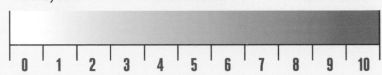

No hay dolor   Dolor moderado   Dolor intenso

0   1   2   3   4   5   6   7   8   9   10

¿Los dolores de cabeza están asociados con?:
Are your headaches associated with:

Sensibilidad a la luz			*Light sensitivity*
Sensibilidad al sonido			*Sound sensitivity*
Náuseas y vomito			*Nausea and vomiting*
Visión borrosa o puntos negros en la visión			*Blurred vision or black spots*
Un tipo particular de comida			*Specific foods*

¿Usted toma medicamentos para el dolor de cabeza?
Do you take any medications for your headaches?

Si usted tiene sus medicamentos aquí, por favor muéstremelos.
If you have your medications with you, please show them to me.

¿Usted tomó sus medicamentos hoy?
Did you take your medications today?

¿Siente rigidez en el cuello desde que el dolor comenzó?
Does your neck feel stiff since the headaches began?

¿Ha tenido usted fiebre o infección recientemente?
Have you had a recent fever or infection?

¿Tiene dolor de cuello o de espalda?
Do you have neck or back pain?

Sírvase indicar cuándo comenzó el dolor.

Please indicate when your pain began.

MINUTOS MINUTES	10	20	30	40	50	60				
HORAS HOURS	2	4	6	8	10	12	14	16	18	20	22
DÍAS DAYS	1	2	3	4	5	6	7	8	9	10	>
SEMANAS WEEKS	1	2	3	4	5	6	7	8	9	10	>
MESES MONTHS	1	2	3	4	5	6	7	8	9	10	>
AÑOS YEARS	1	2	3	4	5	6	7	8	9	10	>

¿El dolor del cuello o la espalda es constante o intermitente?

Is your neck or back pain constant or does it come and go?

 Constante
Constant

 Intermitente
Comes and goes

¿Cómo describiría el dolor?

How would you describe your neck or back pain?

 Sordo
Dull

 Agudo
Sharp

 Como descarga eléctrica
Electric Shock

 Lacerante
Stabbing

¿Se lesionó el cuello o la espalda?
Did you injure your neck or back?

¿El dolor se irradia desde el cuello hasta el brazo?
Does the pain radiate from the neck into your arm?

¿El dolor se irradia desde la espalda hasta la pierna?
Does the pain radiate from your back into your leg?

¿Tiene entumecimiento?
Do you have numbness?

Por favor, señale en su propio cuerpo donde tiene entumecimiento.
Please point on your own body to where you are numb.

¿Siente entumecimiento en el lado izquierdo de su cuerpo,
en el lado derecho o ambos?
Do you feel numbness on the left side of your body, right side
of your body, or both?

 Izquierdo   Derecho   En ambos
Left   Right   Both

¿Siente entumecimiento en la cara, los brazos, las piernas o los tres?
Do you feel numbness in the face, arms, legs, or all three?

 En la cara   En las piernas
Face   Legs

 En los brazos   Los tres
Arms   All three

¿Cuándo comenzó el entumecimiento?
When did the numbness start?

MINUTOS MINUTES	10	20	30	40	50	60				

HORAS HOURS	2	4	6	8	10	12	14	16	18	20	22

DÍAS DAYS	1	2	3	4	5	6	7	8	9	10	>

SEMANAS WEEKS	1	2	3	4	5	6	7	8	9	10	>

MESES MONTHS	1	2	3	4	5	6	7	8	9	10	>

AÑOS YEARS	1	2	3	4	5	6	7	8	9	10	>

¿El entumecimiento inicio de repente?
Did the numbness start suddenly?

¿El entumecimiento es constante o intermitente?
Is the numbness constant or does it come and go?

 Constante Constant   **Intermitente** Comes and goes

¿Tiene ataques convulsivos?
Do you have seizures?

¿Ha tenido ataques convulsivos en el pasado?
Have you had seizures in the past?

NEUROLOGY

76

¿Cuándo fue la última vez que tuvo un ataque?

When was your last seizure?

MINUTOS MINUTES	10	20	30	40	50	60					
HORAS HOURS	2	4	6	8	10	12	14	16	18	20	22
DÍAS DAYS	1	2	3	4	5	6	7	8	9	10	>
SEMANAS WEEKS	1	2	3	4	5	6	7	8	9	10	>
MESES MONTHS	1	2	3	4	5	6	7	8	9	10	>
AÑOS YEARS	1	2	3	4	5	6	7	8	9	10	>

¿Cuánto tiempo hace que tiene ataques?

How long have you had seizures?

SEMANAS WEEKS	1	2	3	4	5	6	7	8	9	10	>
MESES MONTHS	1	2	3	4	5	6	7	8	9	10	>
AÑOS YEARS	1	2	3	4	5	6	7	8	9	10	>

¿Con qué frecuencia tiene ataques?
How often do you have seizures?

 Diariamente
Daily

 1-5 por mes
1-5 per month

 1-5 por semana
1-5 per week

 1-5 por año
1-5 per year

¿Cuánto tiempo duran los ataques?
How long do the seizures last?

30 SEC | **1 MIN** | **15 MIN** | **30 MIN** | **1 HR** | **6 HR** | **12 HR** >

¿Puede anticipar cuando está a punto de tener un ataque?
Can you tell when you are about to have a seizure?

¿Recuerda después que tuvo un ataque?
Do you remember having the seizures?

¿Los ataques hacen que se contorsione o sacuda?
Do the seizures cause you to twitch or jerk?

¿Los ataques hacen que pierda el control de la vejiga o los intestinos?
Do the seizures cause you to lose control of your bladder or bowels?

¿Los ataques hacen que se muerda la lengua o la mejilla?
Do the seizures cause you to bite your tongue or cheek?

¿Después de los ataques se siente confundido o desorientado?
After the seizures do you feel confused or disoriented?

NEUROLOGY

78

¿Después de los ataques se siente cansado?
After the seizures do you feel tired?

¿Después de los ataques se siente enojado o irritado?
After the seizures do you feel angry or upset?

¿Usted toma medicamentos para los ataques?
Do you take medication for your seizures?

¿Tiene dificultades para hablar?
Are you having difficulty speaking?

¿Los problemas del habla comenzaron de repente?
Did the speech problems begin suddenly?

¿Tiene dificultades al tragar?
Do you have difficulty swallowing?

¿Los problemas al tragar comenzaron de repente?
Did the difficulty swallowing begin suddenly?

¿Tiene debilidad?
Do you have weakness?

Por favor, señale en su propio cuerpo donde tiene debilidad.
Please point on your own body where you have weakness.

¿Siente debilidad en el lado izquierdo de su cuerpo, en el lado derecho
o ambos?
Do you feel weakness on the left side of your body, right side of
your body, or both?

 Izquierdo
Left

 Derecho
Right

 En ambos
Both

¿Siente debilidad en los brazos, las piernas o ambos?

Do you feel weak in the arms, legs, or both?

 Brazos
Arms

 Piernas
Legs

 En ambos
Both

¿Cuándo comenzó la debilidad?

When did the weakness start?

MINUTOS	10	20	30	40	50	60					
MINUTES											
HORAS	2	4	6	8	10	12	14	16	18	20	22
HOURS											
DÍAS	1	2	3	4	5	6	7	8	9	10	>
DAYS											
SEMANAS	1	2	3	4	5	6	7	8	9	10	>
WEEKS											
MESES	1	2	3	4	5	6	7	8	9	10	>
MONTHS											
AÑOS	1	2	3	4	5	6	7	8	9	10	>
YEARS											

¿La debilidad inició de repente?

Did the weakness start suddenly?

¿La debilidad es constante o intermitente?

Is the weakness constant or does it come and go?

 Constante
Constant

 Intermitente
Comes and goes

NEUROLOGY

80

Muéstreme sus medicamentos si los tiene aquí.
Show me your medications, if you have them with you.

¿Tiene problemas de la vista?
Do you have vision problems?

¿Ha tenido recientemente pérdida de la visión, visión borrosa o visión doble?
Have you had a recent loss of vision, blurred vision, or double vision?

 Pérdida de la visión
Loss of Vision

 Visión doble
Double Vision

 Visión borrosa
Blurred Vision

¿Cuándo comenzaron los problemas de la visión?
When did the vision trouble start?

MINUTOS MINUTES	10	20	30	40	50	60				
HORAS HOURS	2	4	6	8	10	12	14	16	18	20	22
DÍAS DAYS	1	2	3	4	5	6	7	8	9	10	>
SEMANAS WEEKS	1	2	3	4	5	6	7	8	9	10	>
MESES MONTHS	1	2	3	4	5	6	7	8	9	10	>
AÑOS YEARS	1	2	3	4	5	6	7	8	9	10	>

¿Los problemas de visión comenzaron súbita o gradualmente?
Did the vision trouble start suddenly or gradually?

 De repente
Suddenly

 Gradualmente
Gradually

¿El problema de visión es constante o intermitente?
Is the vision trouble constant or does it come and go?

 Constante
Constant

 Intermitente
Comes and goes

¿El problema de visión es con un ojo o con ambos ojos?
Does the vision trouble involve one eye or both eyes?

 Izquierdo
Left

 Derecho
Right

 En ambos
Both

¿Tiene problemas viendo objetos de cerca, de lejos o ambos?
Do you have trouble seeing objects close, far away, or both?

 De cerca
Close

 De lejos
Far away

 Ambos
Both

¿Normalmente utiliza gafas, contactos o ambos?
Do you normally wear glasses, contact lenses, or both?

 Gafas
Glasses

 Contactos
Contact lenses

 Ambos
Both

82
NEUROLOGIC PROCEDURAL

Por favor, sonría y muéstreme los dientes.
Please smile and show me your teeth.

Por favor, saque la lengua.
Please stick out your tongue.

Por favor, dé su nombre completo y diga donde nació, hablando tan fuerte y claramente como le sea posible.
Please say your full name and where you were born as loudly and as clearly as possible.

Por favor, ponga sus brazos rectos y manténgalos así cuando cierre los ojos.
Please hold your arms out straight and keep them straight when you close your eyes.

Por favor, apriéteme los dedos tan duro como le sea posible.
Please grip my fingers as tight as you can.

Por favor, presione contra mi mano con su pie.
Please push against my hand with your foot.

Por favor, hale su pie contra mi mano.
Please pull your foot up against my hand.

Por favor, encoja los hombros.
Please shrug your shoulders.

Con su dedo índice izquierdo toque mi dedo, luego tóquese la nariz.
With your left index finger touch my finger, then touch your nose.

Con su dedo índice derecho toque mi dedo, luego tóquese la nariz.
With your right index finger touch my finger, then touch your nose.

Doble la rodilla izquierda y coloque el talón del pie izquierdo contra la canilla de la pierna derecha.

Bend your left knee and place your left heel on your right shin.

Doble la rodilla derecha y coloque el talón del pie derecho contra la canilla de la pierna izquierda.

Bend your right knee and place your right heel on your left shin.

Con los ojos cerrados, dígame qué dedo de pie le estoy tocando. ¿Y ahora?

With your eyes closed, tell me what toe I am touching. How about now?

(Testing tactile stimuli to most distal extremities.)

¿Puede levantar la pierna izquierda y mantenerla así diez segundos?

Can you lift and hold your left leg up for me? (hold 10 seconds)

¿Puede levantar la pierna derecha y mantenerla así diez segundos?

Can you lift and hold your right leg up for me? (hold 10 seconds)

Por favor, camine en línea recta brevemente y devuélvase hacia mí.

Please walk in a straight line briefly and then walk back toward me.

Por favor, siga mi dedo/luz con los ojos.

Please follow my finger/light with your eyes.

Por favor, mire mi nariz y señale donde ve mis dedos moverse.

Please look at my nose and point to where you see my fingers wriggling.

84
PAST NEUROLOGIC HISTORY

¿Ha sufrido una apoplejía (derrame) en el pasado?
Have you ever had a stroke in the past?
✓ ✗

¿Cuánto hace que tuvo el derrame?
How long ago did you have the stroke?

DÍAS DAYS	1	2	3	4	5	6	7	8	9	10	>
SEMANAS WEEKS	1	2	3	4	5	6	7	8	9	10	>
MESES MONTHS	1	2	3	4	5	6	7	8	9	10	>
AÑOS YEARS	1	2	3	4	5	6	7	8	9	10	>

¿Usted visita a un neurólogo regularmente?
Do you regularly see a neurologist?
✓ ✗

¿Está tomando algún tipo de medicamento para prevenir derrames?
Are you on any medication to prevent stroke?
✓ ✗

¿Ha tomado sus medicamentos hoy?
Did you take your medication today?
✓ ✗

¿Se le han acabado sus medicamentos?
Have you run out of your medication?
✓ ✗

¿Usted toma?:

Do you take:

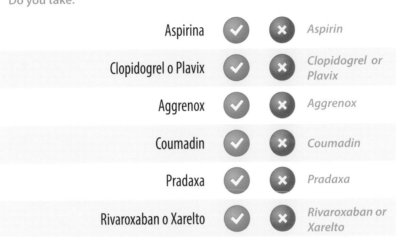

Aspirina	✓	✗	*Aspirin*
Clopidogrel o Plavix	✓	✗	*Clopidogrel or Plavix*
Aggrenox	✓	✗	*Aggrenox*
Coumadin	✓	✗	*Coumadin*
Pradaxa	✓	✗	*Pradaxa*
Rivaroxaban o Xarelto	✓	✗	*Rivaroxaban or Xarelto*

¿Cuándo fue la última vez que tomó sus medicamentos?

When did you last take your medication?

HORAS	2	4	6	8	10	12	14	16	18	20	22
HOURS											

DÍAS	1	2	3	4	5	6	7	8	9	10	>
DAYS											

¿Tiene una receta para medicamentos que todavía no ha obtenido?

Do you have a prescription for medication that you have not filled yet?

¿En los últimos tres meses ha sufrido derrame/AIT?
In the past three months have you had a stroke/TIA?

¿Cuántos derrames/AIT ha sufrido?
How many strokes/TIAs have you had?

  1 2 3 4 5 >

¿Cuándo comenzó el derrame tuvo ataque convulsivo?
Did you have a seizure when the stroke began?

¿Han mejorado los síntomas del derrame?
Are your stroke symptoms getting better?

¿Han desaparecido los síntomas del derrame?
Have your stroke symptoms gone away?

¿En los últimos tres meses ha sufrido un
traumatismo craneal?
In the past three months have you had a head trauma?

¿En los últimos tres meses ha sufrido un infarto?
In the past three months have you had a heart attack?

¿Ha sufrido recientemente de hemorragia
gastrointestinal o del tracto urinario?
Have you had a recent gastrointestinal or urinary tract hemorrhage?

¿Ha tenido una cirugía o un traumatismo en los
últimos 14 días?
Have you had surgery or a recent trauma within the past 14 days?

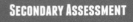
¿Alguna vez ha tenido sangrado o una ruptura arterial en el cerebro?
Have you ever had bleeding or a ruptured artery in the brain?

¿Tiene diabetes?
Do you have diabetes?

¿Fuma cigarrillos o usa tabaco de mascar?
Do you smoke cigarettes/cigars or use chewing tobacco?

¿Usted tiene la presión sanguínea alta?
Do you have high blood pressure?

¿Sufre de palpitaciones cardíacas irregulares?
Do you have an irregular heartbeat?

¿Tiene historial de fibrilación auricular?
Do you have a history of atrial fibrillation?

¿Tiene historial de embolia pulmonar?
Do you have a history of pulmonary embolisms?

¿Tiene historial de coágulos en la sangre?
Do you have a history of blood clots?

¿Tiene historial de meningitis?
Do you have a history of meningitis?

¿Tiene historial de convulciones?
Do you have a history of seizures?

¿Tiene historial de epilepsia?
Do you have a history of epilepsy?

OBSTETRICS

88

Hola, soy un(a) profesional de la salud. No hablo español.

Hello, I am a healthcare professional. I do not speak Spanish.

Respóndame solo sí o no .

Only respond to me "yes" or "no."

ACUTE OBSTETRIC HISTORY

¿Está embarazada?

Are you pregnant?

¿Utilizó recientemente una prueba de embarazo en casa?

Did you recently use a home pregnancy test?

¿Algún médico ha confirmado recientemente
que está embarazada?

Has a physician recently confirmed that you are pregnant?

¿Ya rompió fuente?

Has your water broken?

¿Tiene contracciones?

Are you having contractions?

¿El bebé ya viene ahora?

Is the baby coming now?

¿Siente dolor abdominal?

Do you have abdominal pain?

¿Siente dolor vaginal?

Do you have vaginal pain?

¿Tiene sangrado vaginal?
Do you have vaginal bleeding?

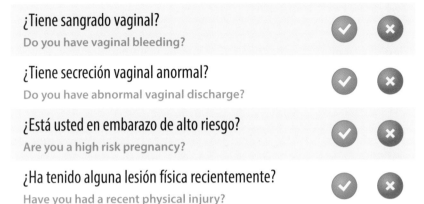

¿Tiene secreción vaginal anormal?
Do you have abnormal vaginal discharge?

¿Está usted en embarazo de alto riesgo?
Are you a high risk pregnancy?

¿Ha tenido alguna lesión física recientemente?
Have you had a recent physical injury?

OBSTETRIC PROCEDURAL

Por favor, cámbiese de ropa y póngase esta bata.
Please change out of your clothes and into this gown.

Por favor, acuéstese en la mesa y ponga los pies en los estribos.
Please lie down on the table and put your feet into the stirrups.

Por favor, baje un poco.
Please move down a bit.

Voy a colocarle suero. Va a sentir una punzada brevemente pero esto es importante hacerlo para poder administrarle medicamentos.
I am going to start an IV. This may sting briefly, but is important so we can give you medication.

Le voy a dar algo de oxígeno mediante el uso de una máscara que va en la cara o dentro la nariz. Puede ser incómodo. Por favor, relájese.
I am going to give you some oxygen either by a mask that goes over you face or up your nose. It may be uncomfortable. Please relax.

OBSTETRICS

90

PAST OBSTETRIC HISTORY

Indique cuántas semanas han pasado desde la última menstruación.

Indicate how many weeks have passed since your last menstrual period.

SEMANAS	1	2	3	4	5	6	7	8	9	10	>
WEEKS											

MESES	1	2	3	4	5	6	7	8	9	10	>
MONTHS											

Indique cuántos meses tiene de embarazo.

Indicate how many months you have been pregnant.

MESES	1	2	3	4	5	6	7	8	9	10	>
MONTHS											

Indique la fecha de su última menstruación.

Please indicate the date of your last menstrual period.

Enero	Mayo	Setiembre	1	2	3	4	5	6	7
January	May	September							
Febrero	Junio	Octubre	8	9	10	11	12	13	14
February	June	October							
			15	16	17	18	19	20	21
Marzo	Julio	Noviembre							
March	July	November	22	23	24	25	26	27	28
Abril	Agosto	Diciembre	29	30	31				
April	August	December							

Indique el número de veces que ha estado embarazada.
Indicate how many times you have been pregnant.

1   2   3   4   5   6   7   8   9   10   >

Indique el número de hijos que tiene.
Indicate how many children you have.

1   2   3   4   5   6   7   8   9   10   >

Indique el número de abortos provocados o abortos espontáneos que haya tenido.
Indicate how many abortions or miscarriages you have had.

1   2   3   4   5   6   7   8   9   10   >

¿Alguna vez ha tenido un embarazo ectópico anterior?
Have you ever had a previous ectopic pregnancy?

¿Ha tenido complicaciones con un embarazo anterior?
Have you had complications with a past pregnancy?

¿Ha tenido un niño con problemas mentales o físicos?
Have you had a child with mental and/or physical handicaps?

¿Ha tenido un niño que nació prematuramente?
Have you had a child that was delivered prematurely?

¿Ha tenido un niño que necesitó cirugía después de haber nacido?
Have you had a child that required surgery after being born?

ONCOLOGY

92

Hola, soy un(a) profesional de la salud. No hablo español.

Hello, I am a healthcare professional. I do not speak Spanish.

Respóndame solo sí o no  .

Only respond to me "yes" or "no."

ACUTE ONCOLOGICAL HISTORY

¿Padece actualmente de cáncer?

Do you currently have cancer?

Por favor señale (en este dibujo de una persona) donde tiene cáncer.

Please point (on this picture of a person) to where you have cancer.

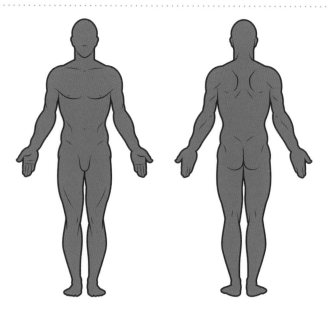

¿Hace metástasis?

Do you have metastases?

¿Cuándo le diagnosticaron el cáncer?
When was your cancer diagnosed?

Enero January	Mayo May	Setiembre September	1	2	3	4	5	6	7
Febrero February	Junio June	Octubre October	8	9	10	11	12	13	14
			15	16	17	18	19	20	21
Marzo March	Julio July	Noviembre November	22	23	24	25	26	27	28
Abril April	Agosto August	Diciembre December	29	30	31				

¿Está recibiendo quimioterapia/radioterapia para el cáncer?

Are you currently receiving chemotherapy/radiation for the cancer?

ACUTE ONCOLOGICAL HISTORY

Voy a acceder a su Porta-cath.
I am going to acces your Porta-cath

Necesito que se ponga esta máscara en la cara.
I need you to put this mask on your face.

Voy a colocarle suero. Va a sentir una punzada brevemente pero esto es importante hacerlo para poder administrarle medicamentos.
I am going to start an IV. This may sting briefly, but is important so we can give you medication.

ONCOLOGY

94

PAST ONCOLOGICAL HISTORY

¿Había tenido cáncer anteriormente?

Have you previously had cancer?

Por favor, señale en este dibujo donde tuvo cáncer.

Please point on this picture where you had cancer.

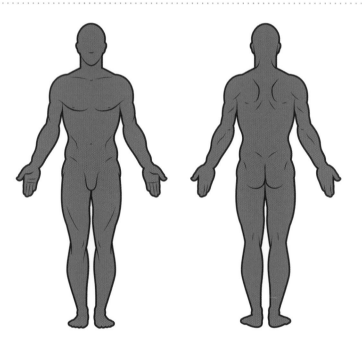

¿Hizo metástasis?

Did you have metastases?

¿Cuándo le diagnosticaron el cáncer?
When was your cancer diagnosed?

Enero January	Mayo May	Setiembre September	
Febrero February	Junio June	Octubre October	
Marzo March	Julio July	Noviembre November	
Abril April	Agosto August	Diciembre December	

1 2 3 4 5 6 7

8 9 10 11 12 13 14

15 16 17 18 19 20 21

22 23 24 25 26 27 28

29 30 31

¿Su cáncer está en remisión?
Is the cancer in remission?

¿Tiene un familiar que tenga cáncer?
Do you have a family member who has cancer?

¿Algún familiar suyo ha fallecido a causa de cáncer?
Do you have a family member who has died due to cancer?

¿Fuma cigarrillos o utiliza productos de tabaco?
Do you smoke cigarettes or use tobacco products?

 Sí
Yes   No
No   Dejé de fumar
I quit

¿Ha tenido un resultado positivo en la prueba de la tuberculosis?
Have you had a positive test for tuberculosis?

Hola, soy un(a) profesional de la salud. No hablo español.

Hello, I am a healthcare professional. I do not speak Spanish.

Respóndame solo sí o no .

Only respond to me "yes" or "no."

ACUTE PEDIATRIC MEDICAL HISTORY

¿Su niño ha tenido recientemente o tiene actualmente
los siguientes síntomas?:

Does your child currently have/recently had the following symptoms:

Dolor abdominal	✓	✕	Abdominal pain
Dolores musculares	✓	✕	Aches
Dolor de espalda	✓	✕	Back pain
Nacidos o abscesos	✓	✕	Boil or abscess
Dolor en los huesos o en las articulaciones	✓	✕	Bone or joint pain
Dolor en el pecho	✓	✕	Chest pain
Escalofríos	✓	✕	Chills
Diarrea	✓	✕	Diarrhea
Dificultad para tragar	✓	✕	Difficulty swallowing

Dificultad para hablar	✓	✕	*Difficulty talking*
Dificultad para caminar y/o moverse	✓	✕	*Difficulty walking/moving*
Mareos	✓	✕	*Dizziness*
Dolor en los oídos	✓	✕	*Earache*
Dolor en los ojos	✓	✕	*Eye pain*
Fiebre	✓	✕	*A fever*
Dolor en los genitales	✓	✕	*Genital pain*
Dolor de cabeza	✓	✕	*A headache*
Problemas de la audición	✓	✕	*Hearing problems*
Irritabilidad	✓	✕	*Irritability*
Dolor en la pierna	✓	✕	*Leg pain*
Náuseas	✓	✕	*Nausea*
Secreción del pezón	✓	✕	*Nipple discharge*
Entumecimiento u hormigueo	✓	✕	*Numbness or tingling*
Sangrado nasal	✓	✕	*A nose bleed*

Problemas psicológicos	✓	✗	*Psychological problems*
Erupción	✓	✗	*Rash*
Sangrado rectal	✓	✗	*Rectal bleeding*
Falta de aire / dificultad para respirar	✓	✗	*Shortness of breath*
Dolor en el hombro	✓	✗	*Shoulder pain*
Cambio de color en la piel	✓	✗	*Skin color change*
Dolor de garganta	✓	✗	*A sore throat*
Dolor de estómago	✓	✗	*Stomach pain*
Hinchazón	✓	✗	*Swelling*
Dificultad para orinar	✓	✗	*Urination difficulty*
Comportamiento violento o agresivo	✓	✗	*Violent or aggressive behavior*
Problemas de visión	✓	✗	*Vision problems*
Vómito	✓	✗	*Vomiting*
Debilidad	✓	✗	*Weakness*

MEDICAL ASSESSMENT TIMELINE

¿Cuándo comenzaron los síntomas de su niño?
When did your child's symptoms begin?

| **MINUTOS** | 10 | 20 | 30 | 40 | 50 | 60 | | | | |
| MINUTES | | | | | | | | | | |

| **HORAS** | 2 | 4 | 6 | 8 | 10 | 12 | 14 | 16 | 18 | 20 | 22 |
| HOURS | | | | | | | | | | | |

| **DÍAS** | 1 | 2 | 3 | 4 | 5 | 6 | 7 | 8 | 9 | 10 | > |
| DAYS | | | | | | | | | | | |

| **MESES** | 1 | 2 | 3 | 4 | 5 | 6 | 7 | 8 | 9 | 10 | > |
| MONTHS | | | | | | | | | | | |

¿Su hijo ha experimentado estos
síntomas previamente?
Has your child's experienced these symptoms previously?

¿Tiene su niño estos síntomas en
repetidas ocasiones?
Does your child have these symptoms repeatedly?

¿Cuándo fue la última vez que tomó los medicamentos que le recetaron?
When did your child last take his or her prescribed medications?

DÍAS   1   2   3   4   5   6   7   8   9   10 >
DAYS

¿Cuándo fue la última vez que comió su niño?
When is the last time your child had food?

DÍAS   1   2   3   4   5   6   7   8   9   10 >
DAYS

¿Su niño puede comer alimentos sólidos sin dificultad?
Can your child eat solid foods without difficulty?
✓ ✗

¿Su niño puede beber líquidos sin dificultad?
Can your child drink liquids without difficulty?
? ✓ ✗

¿Su niño tiene un apetito normal?
Does your child have a normal appetite?
✓ ✗

ACUTE PHYSICAL INJURY HISTORY

¿Su niño está sintiendo dolor?
Is your child in pain?

Por favor, señale en este dibujo donde tiene dolor el niño.
Please point on this picture where your child has pain.

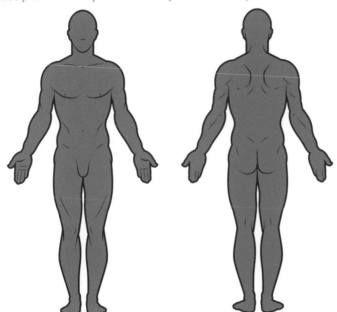

Por favor, indique en esta escala el nivel de dolor de su hijo.
Please point on this scale to rate your child's pain.

No hay dolor   Dolor moderado   Dolor intenso

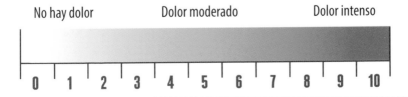

0 1 2 3 4 5 6 7 8 9 10

¿Cuándo fue la última vez que su niño tomó Tylenol o Motrin?
When did your child last have Tylenol or Motrin?

DÍAS   1   2   3   4   5   6   7   8   9   10   >
DAYS

¿Cuánto fue la dosis que le administró?
What was the dose given?   _____ / _____
                                            CUCHARADITAS   **HORA**

¿Cuántas cucharaditas o ml. de medicamento le fueron administradas?
How many teaspoons or milliliters were given?

1   2   3   4   5   6   7   8   9   10   >

PHYSICAL ASSESSMENT TIMELINE

¿Cuándo ocurrió la lesión de su niño?
When did your child's injury occur?

DÍAS   1   2   3   4   5   6   7   8   9   10   >
DAYS

SEMANAS   1   2   3   4   5   6   7   8   9   10   >
WEEKS

MESES   1   2   3   4   5   6   7   8   9   10   >
MONTHS

AÑOS   1   2   3   4   5   6   7   8   9   10   >
YEARS

¿Qué causó esta lesión?
What caused this injury?

✓ **Producto de una agresión**
Assault

✓ **Un accidente de vehículo todo terreno o de moto**
ATV/Motorcycle accident

✓ **Un accidente de carro**
Car accident

✓ **Estrujado o apretado**
Crush

✓ **Una caída**
Fall

✓ **Lesiones deportivas**
Sports injury

✓ **Otro**
Other

✓ **No lo sé.**
I don't know.

¿Su niño perdió el conocimiento?
Did your child lose consciousness?

¿Su hijo estaba usando casco?
Was your child wearing a helmet?

¿Su hijo tenía abrochado el cinturón de seguridad?
Was your child wearing a seatbelt?

¿Se inflaron las bolsas de aire?
Did the airbag deploy?

    El carro no tiene bolsas de aire.
The car does not have airbags.

PEDIATRICS

104

INFANT-SPECIFIC QUESTIONS

¿Su hijo nació al tiempo debido o
a término completo?
Was your child born on time/full term?

Sírvase indicar de cuántas semanas nació su hijo.
Please indicate at how many weeks your child was born.

SEMANAS   30 31 32 33 34 35 36 37 38 39 40 >
WEEKS

¿Se llevó a su niño al salir del hospital o fue necesario
que permaneciera en el hospital más tiempo de lo
esperado después del nacimiento?
Did your child go home from the hospital with you or require
a longer stay in the hospital after birth than expected?

¿Alimenta a su hijo con formula en el biberón, amamantado o ambos?
Is your child bottle/formula fed, breastfed, or both?

 Biberón   **Amamantado**   **Ambos**
Bottle fed   Breastfed   Both

¿Su niño come normalmente?
Is your child eating normal?

¿La orina en los pañales de su hijo es normal?
Is your child having normal urine diapers?

¿El niño hace deposiciones normales?
Is your chid having normal bowel movements?

¿Le salen lágrimas a su niño cuando llora?
Is your child crying tears?

¿Su niño actúa como de costumbre?
Is your child acting like himself?

¿Su niño ha tenido fiebre de más de
100.8 °F (40 °C)?
Has your child had a fever greater than 100.8°F (40°C)?

¿Usted se enfermó de alguna infección
durante el embarazo?
Were you sick with any infections while you were pregnant?

¿Hubo complicaciones con su embarazo o parto?
Were there any complications with your
pregnancy or labor?

¿Cuánto pesó su hijo al nacer?
How much did your child weigh at birth?

LBS	1	2	3	4	5	6	7	8	9	10	>
OZ	1	2	3	4	5	6	7	8	9	10	>
KG	1	2	3	4	5	6	7	8			

106

PEDIATRIC PROCEDURAL

Tengo que colocar una vía intravenosa en su hijo. Esto va a doler.
Por favor, intenta consolar a su hijo.

I need to start an IV on your child. This will hurt.
Please try to comfort your child.

Voy a darle a su hijo una medicación a través de su vía intravenosa.

I am going to give your child some medication through the IV.

Voy a darle a su hijo un poco de medicamento por inyección en la piel.
Puede ser brevemente incómodo.

I am going to give your child some medication by injecting it in the skin.
It may be briefly uncomfortable.

Tengo que colocar una sonda en la vejiga de su hijo. Esto será incómodo.
 Por favor, intenta consolar a su hijo.

I need to place a tube in your child's bladder. This will be uncomfortable.
Please try to comfort you child.

Voy a poner una máscara de oxígeno en la cara de su hijo. Esto
le ayudará a respirar mejor. Esto puede ser incómodo.
Por favor, intenta consolar a su hijo.

I am going to put an oxygen mask on your child's face. This will help him
breathe better. This may be uncomfotable. Please try to comfort your child.

Voy a darle a su hijo un tratamiento de nebulización a través de esta máscara de oxígeno o este tubo. Esto administrará medicamentos que los ayuda a respirar. Esto puede ser incómodo. Por favor, intenta consolar a su hijo.

I am going to give your child a nebulizer treatment through this oxygen mask or pipe. This will deliver medicine to help him breathe. This may be uncomfortable. Please try to comfort your child.

Voy a poner pegatinas en el pecho/brazos/dedos de su hijo. Esto no causará dolor a su hijo.

I am going to put stickers on your child's chest/arms/fingers. This will not hurt your child.

Voy a conseguir la presión arterial de su hijo. Esto puede ser brevemente incómodo. Por favor, consuele a su hijo si se vuelve ansioso.

I am going to get a blood pressure on your child. This may be briefly uncomfortable. Please comfort your child if he becomes anxious.

Voy a suturar la herida de su hijo. Esto va a doler. Por favor, consuele a su hijo. Es importante que se quede quieto.

I am going to suture your child's wound. This will hurt. Please comfort your child. It is important that he stay still.

Voy a poner un yeso o una tablilla en el brazo (s) o pierna (s) de su hijo. Esto puede ser incómodo. Por favor, consuele a su hijo.

I am going to put a cast or splint on your child's arm(s) or leg(s). This may be uncomfortable. Please comfort your child.

PEDIATRICS

108

Voy a poner un yeso o una tablilla en el brazo (s) o pierna (s) de su hijo.
Esto puede ser incómodo. Por favor, consuele a su hijo.

I am going to put a cast or splint on your child's arm(s) or leg(s).
This may be uncomfortable. Please comfort your child.

Voy a llevar a su hijo a hacer una radiografía, tomografía computarizada
o resonancia magnética. Esto no les causará dolor.

I am going to take your child to get an X-Ray, CT, or MRI scan.
This will not hurt him.

Por favor, quédese aquí. Volveremos en breve.

Please stay here. We will return shortly.

Puede venir con nosotros.

You may come with us.

Tengo que meter este hisopo de algodón en la nariz de su hijo
o en su garganta. Este será brevemente incómodo.

I need to stick this cotton swab up your child's nose or in his throat.
This will be briefly uncomfortable.

Tengo que obtener una muestra de heces de su hijo.

I need to obtain a stool sample from your child.

Tengo que obtener una muestra de orina de su hijo.

I need to obtain a urine sample from your child.

Past Pediatric History

Allergies

¿Su niño tiene alergia a algún medicamento?
Does your child have allergies to any medications?

¿Su niño tiene alergia a alguna comida?
Does your child have allergies to foods?

¿Sufre su niño de alergias estacionales?
Does your child have seasonal allergies?

¿Su hijo es alérgico al látex?
Is your child allergic to latex?

Medications

¿Su niño toma medicamentos en forma regular?
Does you child take medications on a regular basis?

¿Le han dado al niño algún medicamento hoy?
Have you given your child any medications today?

Si tiene los medicamentos del niño, por favor muéstremelos.
If you have them with you, please show me your child's medications.

¿Se le han acabado los medicamentos del niño?
Have you run out of your child's medication?

PEDIATRICS

MEDICAL CONDITIONS

¿Su niño tiene o ha tenido historial de?:

Does your child have a history of:

ADHD (déficit de atención e hiperactividad)	✓	✗	ADHD
ODD (trastorno negativista desafiante)	✓	✗	ODD
Trastornos del espectro autista	✓	✗	Autistic spectrum disorders
Ingestión accidental	✓	✗	Accidental ingestions
Asma	✓	✗	Asthma
Fibrilación auricular	✓	✗	Atrial fibrillation
Trastorno de coagulación de la sangre	✓	✗	Blood clotting disorder
Bronquitis	✓	✗	Bronchitis
Cáncer	✓	✗	Cancer
Parálisis cerebral	✓	✗	Cerebral palsy
Varicela	✓	✗	Chicken pox
Insuficiencia renal crónica	✓	✗	Chronic renal failure
Complicaciones de la circuncisión	✓	✗	Circumcision complications

Crup	✓	✗	Croup
Cortes, heridas, contusiones o heridas que no se han curado	✓	✗	Cuts, wounds, abrasions, or sores that haven't healed
Problemas dentales	✓	✗	Dental problems
Condiciones dermatológicas	✓	✗	Dermatological conditions
Diabetes Mellitus Tipo 1	✓	✗	Diabetes mellitus Type 1 (IDDM)
Diabetes Mellitus Tipo 2	✓	✗	Diabetes mellitus Type 2
Enfisema	✓	✗	Emphysema
Disfunción del sistema endocrino	✓	✗	Endocrine system dysfunction
Epiglotitis	✓	✗	Epiglottitis
Problemas genitales (hombres)	✓	✗	Genital problems (Male)
Problemas ginecológicos	✓	✗	Gynecological problems
VIH/SIDA	✓	✗	HIV/AIDs
Problemas de la audición	✓	✗	Hearing problems
Hemofilia	✓	✗	Hemophilia
Hyperbilirubinemia	✓	✗	Hyperbilirubinemia

Alta presión	✓	✗	High blood pressure
Enfermedad de Hirschsprung	✓	✗	Hirschsprung's disease
Hipospadias	✓	✗	Hypospadias
Problemas del sistema inmunológico	✓	✗	Immune system conditions
Problemas intestinales	✓	✗	Intestinal conditions
Invaginación intestinal	✓	✗	Intussusception
Artritis juvenil reumatoidea	✓	✗	Junior rheumatoid arthritis
Síndrome de Kawasaki	✓	✗	Kawasaki's disease
Meningitis	✓	✗	Meningitis
Enterocolitis necrotizante	✓	✗	Necrotizing enterocolitis
Osteogénesis imperfecta	✓	✗	Osteogenesis imperfecta
Trasplante de órganos	✓	✗	Organ transplant
Agresión física o sexual	✓	✗	Physical/ sexual assault
Enterobiasis	✓	✗	Pinworms
Neumonía	✓	✗	Pneumonia
Problemas psiquiátricos	✓	✗	Psychiatric conditions
Fisioterapia para una lesión	✓	✗	Physical therapy for an injury

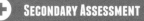
Cirugía reciente	✓	✗	*Recent surgery*
El VSR/Bronquiolitis	✓	✗	*RSV/Bronchiolitis*
Escabiosis	✓	✗	*Scabies*
Escoliosis	✓	✗	*Scoliosis*
Convulsiones o problemas neurológicos	✓	✗	*Seizures/neurological conditions*
Convulsiones febriles	✓	✗	*Febrile seizures*
Crisis drepanocítica	✓	✗	*Sickle cell crises*
Espina bífida	✓	✗	*Spina bifida*
Estado postoperatorio de la amigdalectomía y adenoidectomía	✓	✗	*Status post tonsillectomy and adenoidectomy bleed*
Candidiasis bucal / infecciones causadas por levaduras candidas	✓	✗	*Thrush/yeast infections*
Fístulas transesofágicas	✓	✗	*Transesophageal fistulas*
Úlceras o problemas estomacales	✓	✗	*Ulcers or stomach conditions*
Problemas de la vista	✓	✗	*Vision problems*

¿Ha vacunado a su niño contra
la hepatitis B (HepB)?

Has your child had his Hepatitis B (HepB) vaccine?

¿Ha vacunado a su niño contra
la hepatitis A (HepA)?

Has your child had his Hepatitis A (HepA) vaccine?

¿Ha vacunado a su niño contra el tétano
y contra la tos ferina (DTPA)?

Has your child had his Diphtheria and

tetanus toxoids and acellular pertussis vaccine (DTaP)?

¿Ha vacunado a su niño contra el rotavirus (RV)?

Has your child had his Rotavirus vaccine (RV)?

¿Ha vacunado a su niño contra el virus
del polio?

Has your child had his inactivated poliovirus vaccine (IPV)?

¿Su niño ha recibido la vacuna conjugada contra
la Haemophilus influenza tipo b (Hib/HbCV)?

Has your child had his Haemophilus Influenzae Type B

conjugate vaccine (Hib/HbCV) Immunization?

¿Ha vacunado a su niño contra el
resfriado (estacional)?

Has your child had his influenza vaccine (seasonal)?

Su niño ha recibido la vacuna antimeningocócica conjugada, tetravalente (MCV4)?

Has your child had his Meningococcal conjugate vaccine, quadrivalent (MCV4) vaccine?

¿Su niño ha recibido la vacuna triple vírica (sarampión, paperas y rubéola)?

Has your child had his MMR (measles, mumps, and rubella) vaccine?

¿Ha vacunado a su niño contra el neumococo (VCN)?

Has your child had his pneumococcal vaccine (PCV)?

¿Ha vacunado a su niño contra el virus del papiloma humano (VPH)?

Has your child had his human papillomavirus vaccine (HPV)?

¿Se le ha hecho a su niño la prueba de tuberculina (PPD)?

Has your child had his tuberculin skin test (PPD)?

¿Arrojó resultado positivo o negativo?

Was it negative or positive?

¿Su niño ha recibido la vacuna contra el tétano en los últimos 10 años?

Has your child had a tetanus vaccine within the last 10 years?

¿Su niño ha recibido la vacuna contra el resfriado en el último año?

Has your child had an influenza vaccine within the last year?

¿La vacuna de su hijo contra la neumonía neumocócica está al día?

Is your child's pneumococcal pneumonia vaccine up to date?

Por favor, anote el nombre del médico de cabecera de su hijo.

Please write the name of your child's primary care physician or provider.

 ### No tengo médico de cabecera o proveedor médico.

I don't have a primary care physician or provider.

Por favor, anote la dirección del médico de cabecera de su hijo.

Please write the address of your child's primary care physician or provider.

Calle (Street)   Apartamento (Apt. #)

Ciudad (City)   Estado (State)   Código Postal (ZIP)

Por favor, anote el número de teléfono del médico de cabecera de su hijo.

Please write the phone number of your child's primary care physician.

(_____) _____ – _____

TB SCREENING

¿Su niño ha tenido tos prolongada durante 3 semanas o más?
Has your child had a prolonged cough for 3 weeks or more?

¿Su niño ha tenido pérdida de peso inexplicable?
Has your child had unexplained weight loss?

¿Su niño ha tenido fiebre y escalofríos recientemente?
Has your child had a recent fever/chills?

¿Su niño ha tenido sangre en el esputo?
Has your child had any blood in the sputum?

¿Su niño ha sido indigente o ha estado
sin hogar alguna vez?
Has your child ever been homeless?

¿Su niño tiene o ha tenido historial de tuberculosis
activa en algún momento?
Does your child have a history of active tuberculosis now or at anytime?

¿Su niño ha arrojado resultados positivos en la prueba
contra la tuberculosis en los últimos 2 años?
Has your child had a positive tuberculosis test within the past 2 years?

¿Su niño tiene bomba de insulina?
Does your child have an insulin pump?

¿Su niño tiene instrucciones anticipadas?
Does your child have an advance directive?

¿Desea asistencia para redactar instrucciones anticipadas para su hijo?
Do you want assistance with an advance directive for your child?

¿Está usted seguro en el entorno de su casa?
Are you safe in your home environment?

¿Desea que nos pongamos en contacto con cuidado pastoral?
Do you want us to contact Pastoral Care?

¿Desea que nos pongamos en contacto con Servicios Sociales?
Do you want us to contact Social Services?

¿Desea que nos pongamos en contacto con un intérprete?
Do you want us to contact an interpreter?

¿Su niño tiene historial de deterioro en la capacidad cognitiva?
Does your child have a history of impaired cognitive ability?

¿Su hijo es un peligro para sí mismo o los demás?
Is your child a danger to self or others?

¿Su niño tiene historial de fuga?
Does your child have a history of running away from home?

¿Su niño expresa su intención de irse?
Does your child verbalize an attempt to leave?

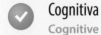
¿Su niño tiene alguna de las siguientes barreras de aprendizaje?

Does your child have any of the following learning barriers?

- ✓ **Cognitiva**
  Cognitive
- ✓ **Educación**
  Education
- ✓ **Audición**
  Hearing

- ✓ **Aprendizaje**
  Learning
- ✓ **Otro**
  Other
- ✗ **No**
  No

¿Su niño tiene alguna de las siguientes necesidades especiales?

Does your child have any of the following special needs?

- ✓ **Cultural**
  Cultural
- ✓ **Emocional**
  Emotional
- ✓ **Aflicción**
  Grief
- ✓ **Pérdida**
  Loss
- ✓ **Personal**
  Personal

- ✓ **Religiosa**
  Religious
- ✓ **Social**
  Social
- ✓ **Física**
  Physical
- ✓ **Otro**
  Other
- ✗ **No**
  No

PEDIATRIC SCREENINGS ·

120

¿Cuándo fue la última fecha en la que su hijo fue visto
por última vez normal/bien?

When was the last date your child seemed normal/well?

Enero January	Mayo May	Setiembre September	1	2	3	4	5	6	7
Febrero February	Junio June	Octubre October	8	9	10	11	12	13	14
			15	16	17	18	19	20	21
Marzo March	Julio July	Noviembre November	22	23	24	25	26	27	28
Abril April	Agosto August	Diciembre December	29	30	31				

¿Cuándo fue la última vez (hoy) en la que su hijo fue visto
por última vez normal/bien?

When was the last time (today) your child seemed normal/well?

AM	1	2	3	4	5	6	7	8	9	10	11	12
PM	1	2	3	4	5	6	7	8	9	10	11	12

¿Está su hijo expuesto al humo de tabaco?

Is your child exposed to tobacco smoke?

?

Hola, soy un(a) profesional de la salud. No hablo español.

Hello, I am a healthcare professional. I do not speak Spanish.

Respóndame solo sí o no .

Only respond to me "yes" or "no."

ACUTE PSYCHIATRIC/PSYCHOLOGICAL HISTORY

¿Se siente triste o deprimido?

Do you feel sad or depressed?

¿Tiene la sensación de querer hacerse daño
físicamente a si mismo u a otras personas?

Do you have feelings of wanting to physically hurt yourself or others?

¿Tiene planeado hacerse daño físicamente a
si mismo u a otras personas?

Do you have a plan to physically hurt yourself or others?

¿Padece actualmente de ansiedad?

Do you currently have anxiety?

¿Se preocupa constantemente?

Do you worry constantly?

¿Teme que alguien le haga daño?

Are you afraid of someone harming you?

¿Tiene sentimientos abrumadores de culpa?

Do you feel overwhelming guilt?

PSYCHIATRY/PSYCHOLOGY

122

PSYCHIATRIC/PSYCHOLOGICAL PROCEDURAL

Por favor, cámbiese de ropa y póngase esta bata.
Please change out of your clothes and into this gown.

Por favor, tómese este medicamento con agua.
Please take this oral medication and swallow with water.

Vamos a administrarle un medicamento por vía intravenosa
o intramuscular.
We are going to give you some medication through your IV or
into your muscles.

PAST PSYCHIATRIC/PSYCHOLOGICAL HISTORY

¿Bebe más de cinco bebidas alcohólicas al día?
Do you drink more than five alcoholic drinks a day?

 Sí
Yes

 No
No

 Dejé el trago
I quit

Por favor, indique el tipo de bebida alcohólica que normalmente consume.
Please indicate type of alcohol you normally drink.

 Cerveza
Beer

 Whiskey
Whiskey

 Vodka
Vodka

 Bourbon
Bourbon

 Vino
Wine

 Otra
Other

 Ginebra
Gin

¿Fuma cigarrillos o utiliza productos de tabaco?
Do you smoke cigarettes or use tobacco products?

 Sí
Yes

 No
No

 Dejé de fumar
I quit

¿Utiliza alguna droga ilícita o medicamentos que no fueron prescritos para usted?
Do you use any illicit drugs/medications that were not prescribed to you?

 Sí
Yes

 No
No

 Dejé las drogas
I quit

Por favor, indique qué tipo de drogas utiliza.
Please indicate what type of drugs you use.

 Cocaína
Cocaine

 Éxtasis
Ecstasy

 Heroína
Heroin

 LSD/ "ácido"
LSD/"acid"

 Marihuana
Marijuana

 Metanfetaminas
Methamphetamines

Otra
Other

Por favor, indique de qué forma usa estas drogas.
Please indicate in which form you use these drugs.

✓ **Inyectada por vía intravenosa**
Inject intravenously

✓ **Introducida por vía rectal**
Insert rectally

✓ **Fumada**
Smoke

✓ **Aspirada por la nariz**
Snort

✓ **Por vía oral en forma de píldora**
Swallow in pill form

✓ **Otra**
Other

¿Ha sufrido antes de maltrato físico?
Have you been physically abused before?

¿Ha sufrido antes de abuso sexual?
Have you been sexually abused before?

¿Ha sufrido antes de abuso emocional?
Have you been emotionally abused before?
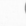

¿Usted toma medicamentos para la ansiedad?
Do you take medication for anxiety?

 Sí, regularmente
Yes, regularly.

No
No

 Sí, pero no soy constante.
Yes, but I am not consistent.

Un médico me ha recetado medicamentos para la ansiedad pero no los tomo.
I have been prescribed medication for anxiety by a physician but do not take it.

¿Usted toma medicamentos para el trastorno bipolar?
Do you take medication for Bi-Polar Disorder?

 Sí, regularmente
Yes, regularly.

No
No

Sí, pero no soy constante.
Yes, but I am not consistent.

 Un médico me ha recetado medicamentos para el trastorno bipolar pero no los tomo.
I have been prescribed medication for Bi-Polar Disorder by a physician but do not take it.

¿Usted toma medicamentos para la depresión?

Do you take medication for depression?

 Sí, regularmente
Yes, regularly.

 No
No

 Sí, pero no soy constante.
Yes, but I am not consistent.

 Un médico me ha recetado medicamentos para la depresión pero no los tomo.
I have been prescribed medication for depression by a physician but do not take it.

¿Usted toma medicamentos para la esquizofrenia?

Do you take medication for schizophrenia?

 Sí, regularmente
Yes, regularly.

 No
No

 Sí, pero no soy constante.
Yes, but I am not consistent.

 Un médico me ha recetado medicamentos para la esquizofrenia pero no los tomo.
I have been prescribed medication for schizophrenia by a physician but do not take it.

ACUTE PULMONOLOGICAL HISTORY

¿Tiene dificultad para respirar?
Do you have shortness of breath?

¿Cuándo comenzó la dificultad para respirar?
When did your shortness of breath begin?

DÍAS   1   2   3   4   5   6   7   8   9   10   >
DAYS

¿Siente dolor en el pecho?
Do you have chest pain?

Por favor, señale sobre su propio pecho exactamente donde siente dolor.
Please point on your own chest to where you have chest pain.

¿Le duele respirar?
Does it hurt to breathe?

¿Utiliza un inhalador de dosis medida (IDM) en casa?
Do you use a metered dose inhaler (MDI) at home?

   Sí
         Yes

   Sí, pero se me acabó medicamento.
         Yes, but I ran out of medication.

   No
         No

¿Cuándo fue la última vez que usó el inhalador de dosis medida (IDM)?

When was the last time you used your metered dose inhaler (MDI)?

DÍAS   1   2   3   4   5   6   7   8   9   10   >
DAYS

¿Cuántas veces ha usado el inhalador de dosis medida (IDM) hoy?

How many times have you used your metered dose inhaler (MDI) today?

1   2   3   4   5   6   7   8   9   10   >

¿El inhalador de dosis medida le sirve cuando siente que le falta el aire?

Did the metered dose inhaler help your shortness of breath?

 Sí
Yes

 No
No

Un poco
A little

¿Usted utiliza un espaciador o cámara con el inhalador
de dosis medida (IDM)?

Do you use a spacer/chamber with your metered dose inhaler (MDI)?

 Sí
Yes

No
No

Sí, a veces
Yes, sometimes

¿Tiene congestión nasal?

Do you have nasal congestion?

¿Tiene tos?
Do you have a cough?

¿Tiene esputo al toser?
Are you coughing up any sputum?

¿De qué color es el esputo?
What color is your sputum?

 Marrón
Brown

 Rojo
Red

 Verde
Green

 Amarillo
Yellow

 Negro
Black

¿Hay sangre presente en el esputo?
Is there any blood in your sputum?

¿Alguna vez ha sido encarcelado o ha estado en una prisión?
Have you ever been incarcerated/in prison?

¿Ha estado expuesto a la tuberculosis?
Have you been exposed to tuberculosis?

¿La tos cambia al cambiar el clima?
Does your cough change with the weather?

PULMONOLOGIC PROCEDURAL

Por favor, quítese la ropa y póngase esta bata.
Please change out of your clothes and into this gown.

Necesito escuchar sus pulmones. Por favor, respire normalmente.
I need to listen to your lungs. Please breathe normally.

Necesito escuchar sus pulmones. Por favor, respire profundo y despacio.
I need to listen to your lungs. Please breathe deeply and slowly.

Le voy a administrar oxígeno por la nariz. Esto puede ser un poco incómodo.
I am going to give you oxygen through your nose.
This may be mildly uncomfortable.

Le voy a dar oxígeno a través de esta máscara que se coloca sobre la boca y la nariz. Esto puede ser un poco incómodo.
I am going to give you oxygen through this mask that will will go over your mouth and nose. This may be mildly uncomfortable.

Le voy a colocar un ventilador de presión positiva en modo CPAP o uno de ventilación no invasiva en modo BiPAP. Se siente como si usted hubiera sacado la cabeza por la ventana de un carro en movimiento y será brevemente incómodo.
I am going to put you on a CPAP or BiPAP. It will feel like your head is outside the window of a moving car and will be uncomfortable for a little bit.

Le voy a administrar medicamento mediante un inhalador que calibra la dosis. Esto no le va a doler.

I am going to give you medication through a metered dose inhaler. This will not hurt.

 Por favor, exhale totalmente.
Please exhale completely.

 Por favor, inhale profundamente.
Please inhale deeply.

Le voy a administrar medicamento mediante un nebulizador. Esto no le va a doler. Por favor, inhale lenta y profundamente.

I am going to give you medication through a nebulizer. This will not hurt. Please inhale slowly and deeply.

PAST PULMONOLOGICAL HISTORY

¿Tiene historial de asma?
Do you have a history of asthma?

 Sí
Yes

 No
No

 Sí, pero solo cuando niño.
Yes, but only as a child.

¿Alguna vez lo han entubado (un tubo en la garganta para ayudarle a respirar) debido a su asma?
Have you ever been intubated (a tube down your throat to help you breathe) because of your asthma?

¿Cuántas veces ha sido entubado?

How many times have you been intubated?

1   2   3   4   5   6   7   8   9   10   >

¿Usted utiliza un espaciador o cámara con el inhalador de dosis medida (IDM)?

Do you use a spacer/chamber with your metered dose inhaler (MDI)?

 Sí
Yes

 No
No

 No, pero antes tenía.
No, but I used to.

¿Usted toma corticosteroides para el asma?

Do you take corticosteroids for your asthma?

 Sí
Yes

 No
No

 No, pero usaba antes.
No, but I used to.

¿Ha estado en la unidad de cuidados intensivos (UCI) por causa del asma?

Have you been in the intensive care unit (ICU) for your asthma?

¿Cuántas veces ha sido internado en un hospital debido al asma?

How many times have you been admitted to a hospital due to your asthma?

1   2   3   4   5   6   7   8   9   10   >

¿Tiene historial de?:

Do you have a history of:

Fibrilación auricular	✔	✖	*Atrial fibrillation*
Bronquitis	✔	✖	*Bronchitis*
Enfermedad pulmonar obstructiva crónica	✔	✖	*Chronic obstructive pulmonary disease*
Insuficiencia cardíaca congestiva	✔	✖	*Congestive heart failure*
Enfisema	✔	✖	*Emphysema*
Neumonía	✔	✖	*Pneumonia*
Edema pulmonar	✔	✖	*Pulmonary edema*
Embolia pulmonar	✔	✖	*Pulmonary embolisms*
Tuberculosis	✔	✖	*Tuberculosis*

¿Tiene implantado un marcapasos o desfibrilador?

Do you have an implanted pacemaker/defibrillator?

¿Lo han vacunado a usted contra la Hepatitis B (HepB)?

Have you had your Hepatitis B (HepB) vaccine?

¿Lo han vacunado a usted contra la Hepatitis A (HepA)?

Have you had your Hepatitis A (HepA) vaccine?

¿Lo han vacunado a usted contra la difteria, el tétano y contra la tos ferina (DTPA)?

Have you had your Diphtheria and tetanus toxoids and acellular pertussis vaccine (DTaP)?

¿Lo han vacunado contra el rotavirus (RV)?

Have you had your Rotavirus vaccine (RV)?

¿Lo han vacunado contra el poliovirus (IPV)?

Have you had your inactivate poliovirus vaccine (IPV)?

¿Le han aplicado la vacuna conjugada contra la Haemophilus influenzae tipo b (Hib/HbCV)?

Have you had your Haemophilus Influenzae Type B conjugate vaccine (Hib/HbCV) Immunization?

¿Lo han vacunado contra el resfriado (estacional)?

Have you had your influenza vaccine (seasonal)?

¿Le han aplicado la vacuna antimeningocócica conjugada, tetravalente (MCV4)?
Have you had your Meningococcal conjugate vaccine, quadrivalent (MCV4) vaccine?

¿Le han aplicado la vacuna triple vírica (sarampión, paperas y rubéola)?
Have you had your MMR (measles, mumps, and rubella) vaccine?

¿Lo han vacunado contra el neumococo (VCN)?
Have you had your Pneumococcal vaccine (PCV)?

¿Lo han vacunado contra el virus del papiloma humano (VPH)?
Have you had your human papillomavirus vaccine (HPV)?

¿Le han hecho la prueba de tuberculina (PPD)?
Have you had your tuberculin skin test (PPD)?

¿Arrojó resultado positivo o negativo?
Was it negative or positive?

¿Se ha vacunado contra el tétano en los últimos 10 años?
Have you had a tetanus vaccine within the last 10 years?

¿Se ha vacunado contra el resfriado en el último año?
Have you had an influenza vaccine within the last year?

¿La vacuna contra la neumonía neumocócica está al día?

Is your pneumococcal pneumonia vaccine up to date?

Por favor, anote el nombre de su médico de cabecera.

Please write the name of your primary care physician or provider.

 No tengo médico de cabecera o proveedor médico.
I don't have a primary care physician or provider.

Por favor, anote la dirección de su médico de cabecera.

Please write the address of your primary care physician or provider.

Calle (Street)   Apartamento (Apt. #)

Ciudad (City)   Estado (State)   Código Postal (ZIP)

Por favor, anote el número de teléfono de su médico de cabecera.

Please write the phone number of your primary care physician or provider.

(_____) _____ – _____

TB SCREENING

¿Ha tenido usted tos prolongada por 3 semanas o más?
Have you had a prolonged cough for 3 weeks or more?

¿Ha tenido pérdida de peso inexplicable?
Have you had unexplained weight loss?

¿Ha tenido usted fiebre y escalofríos recientemente?
Have you had a recent fever/chills?

¿Ha visto usted sangre en el esputo?
Have you had any blood in your sputum?

¿Ha sido alguna vez indigente o ha estado sin hogar?
Have you ever been homeless?

¿Tiene o ha tenido historial de tuberculosis activa en algún momento?
Do you have a history of active tuberculosis now or at anytime?

¿Ha arrojado resultados positivos en la prueba contra la tuberculosis en los últimos 2 años?
Have you had a positive tuberculosis test within the past 2 years?

¿Tiene bomba de insulina?
Do you have an insulin pump?

¿Tiene redactado un documento de instrucciones anticipadas?
Do you have an advance directive?

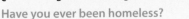

¿Desea asistencia para redactar instrucciones anticipadas?
Do you want assistance with an advance directive?

¿Está usted seguro en el entorno de su casa?
Are you safe in your home environment?

¿Desea que nos pongamos en contacto con cuidado pastoral?
Do you want us to contact Pastoral Care?

¿Desea que nos pongamos en contacto con Servicios Sociales?
Do you want us to contact Social Services?

¿Desea que nos pongamos en contacto con un intérprete?
Do you want us to contact an interpreter?

¿Desea que nosotros ó el intérprete contacte a un pariente?
Do you want us/the interpreter to contact a family member?

Este familiar es:
This family member is a:

 Esposo(a)
Spouse

 Hijo(a)
Child

 Padre o Madre
Parent

 Otro pariente
Other relative

Anote el número de teléfono del pariente:
Please write down their phone number: (_____) _____-_____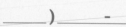

FOR CAREGIVER/FAMILY/WITNESS

¿El paciente tiene un historial de confusión o la demencia?
Does the patient have a history of confusion or dementia?

¿El paciente tiene historial de deterioro en la capacidad cognitiva?
Does the patient have a history of impaired cognitive ability?

¿El paciente es un peligro para sí mismo o los demás?
Is the patient a danger to self or others?

¿El paciente tiene historial de fuga?
Does the patient have a history of wandering off?

¿El paciente expresa su intención de irse?
Does the patient verbalize an attempt to leave?

¿El paciente tiene alguna de las siguientes necesidades especiales?
Does the patient have any of the following special needs?

Cultural
Cultural

Religiosa
Religious

Emocional
Emotional

Social
Social

Aflicción
Grief

Otro
Other

Pérdida
Loss

No lo sé.
I don't know.

Personal
Personal

¿El paciente tiene alguna de las siguientes barreras de aprendizaje?
Does the patient have any of the following learning barriers?

✓ **Cognitiva**
Cognitive

✓ **Aprendizaje**
Learning

✓ **Educación**
Education

✓ **Otro**
Other

✓ **Audición**
Hearing

✓ **No lo sé.**
I don't know.

¿Cuándo fue la última fecha en la que el paciente fue visto por última vez normal/bien?
When was the last date the patient seemed normal/well?

Enero January	Mayo May	Setiembre September	1	2	3	4	5	6	7
Febrero February	Junio June	Octubre October	8	9	10	11	12	13	14
			15	16	17	18	19	20	21
Marzo March	Julio July	Noviembre November	22	23	24	25	26	27	28
Abril April	Agosto August	Diciembre December	29	30	31				

¿Cuándo fue la última vez (hoy) en la que el paciente fue visto por última vez normal/bien?
When was the last time (today) the patient seemed normal/well?

AM	1	2	3	4	5	6	7	8	9	10	11	12
PM	1	2	3	4	5	6	7	8	9	10	11	12

BEDSIDE

Aquí está el botón luminoso para llamar.
Oprima este botón si necesita mi ayuda.
Here is your call light/button. Press this button if you need my help.

Aquí está su orinal o pato (cuña).
Here is your urinal or bed pan.

DIAGNOSTICS

Le voy a tomar la temperatura por vía oral. Por favor, abra la boca
y levante la lengua. Este procedimiento no es doloroso.
I am going to take your oral temperature. Please open your mouth
and lift up your tongue. This procedure will not hurt.

Le voy a tomar la temperatura timpánica. Voy a pegarle un
pequeño dispositivo en el oído. Este procedimiento no es doloroso.
I am going to take your tympanic temperature. I will stick a small device
in your ear. This procedure will not hurt.

Voy a usar un doppler. Por favor, quédese quieto durante
el procedimiento. Este procedimiento no es doloroso.
I am going to use a doppler. Please stay still during the procedure.
This procedure will not hurt.

Un intérprete estará aquí pronto.

An interpreter will be here shortly.

Sé que muchas cosas están pasando alrededor de usted.
No tenga miedo. Todos estamos aquí para ayudarlo.

I know that a lot of things may be happening around you.
Do not be afraid. We are all here to help you.

Tengo que ponerle un collarín cervical alrededor del cuello
para proteger la columna vertebral de una lesión mayor.
Esto puede ser incómodo.

I need to put a cervical collar around your neck to protect your spine
from further injury. This may be uncomfortable.

Tengo que inmovilizarlo sobre este respaldo para proteger la
columna de una lesión. Esto puede ser incómodo.

I need to immobilize your body on a backboard to protect your spine
from injury. This may be uncomfortable.

Le voy a enyesar la extremidad lesionada. Esto puede ser doloroso.

I am going to put a cast on your injured limb. This may be painful.

Lo siento pero no puedo darle líquidos.

I am sorry but I cannot give you liquids.

Lo siento pero no puedo darle comida.

I am sorry but I cannot give you food.

Regresaré en unos momentos para ver cómo se siente.

I will return shortly to check up on you.

Sígame por favor.
Please follow me.

Quédese quieto por favor.
Please be still.

Por favor, relájese.
Please relax.

Estoy aquí para ayudarle.
I am here to help.

Voy a llevarlo a su habitación.
I am going to take you to your room.

Por favor, sígame.
Please follow me.

Por favor, siéntese.
Please sit down.

Por favor, acuéstese.
Please lie down.

Por favor, póngase de pie.
Please stand up.

Por favor, camine hacia mi.
Please walk toward me.

Por favor, métase a la cama.
Please get in bed.

Por favor, siéntese en la silla de ruedas.
Please sit in the wheelchair.

Le voy a administrar oxígeno por la nariz. Esto puede ser un poco incómodo.

I am going to give you oxygen through your nose.
This may be mildly uncomfortable.

Le voy a dar oxígeno a través de esta máscara que se coloca sobre la boca y la nariz. Esto puede ser un poco incómodo.

I am going to give you oxygen through this mask that will will go over your mouth and nose. This may be mildly uncomfortable.

Le voy a colocar un ventilador de presión positiva en modo CPAP o uno de ventilación no invasiva en modo BiPAP. Se siente como si usted hubiera sacado la cabeza por la ventana de un carro en movimiento y será brevemente incómodo.

I am going to put you on a CPAP or BiPAP. It will feel like your head is outside the window of a moving car and will be uncomfortable for a little bit.

Le voy a administrar medicamento mediante un inhalador que calibra la dosis. Este procedimiento no es doloroso.

I am going to give you medication through metered dose inhaler. This will not hurt.

Por favor, exhale totalmente.

Please exhale completely.

Por favor, inhale profundamente.

Please inhale deeply.

Le voy a administrar medicamento mediante un nebulizador. Esto no le va a doler. Por favor, inhale lenta y profundamente.

I am going to give you medication through a nebulizer. This will not hurt. Please inhale slowly and deeply.

Voy a colocarle suero. Sentirá dolor brevemente pero esto es importante hacerlo para poder administrarle medicamentos.

I am going to start an IV. This will hurt briefly but is important so we can give you medication.

Le voy a administrar medicamento en el suero.
Tal vez le incomode brevemente.

I am going to give you some medication through your IV. You may feel uncomfortable for a little bit.

Le voy a administrar medicamento con esta jeringa. Tal vez le arda o se sienta incomodo brevemente pero la sensación pasa rápido.

I am going to give you some medication with this needle. This may sting or feel uncomfortable for a little bit but the feeling will pass quickly.

Le voy a sacar una muestra de sangre. Tal vez le incomode brevemente.

I am going to draw a blood sample. It may feel a little uncomfortable.

Voy a colocarle un catéter central. Va a sentir dolor.

I am going to start a central line. This will hurt.

Voy a ganar acceso al catéter central. No va a sentir dolor.

I am going to access your central line. This will not hurt.

Voy a colocarle un catéter central de inserción periférica. Va a sentir dolor.

I am going to start a PICC line. This will hurt.

Voy a colocarle un portacath. Va a sentir dolor.

I am going to start a portacath. This will hurt.

Voy a ganar acceso al portacath. No va a sentir dolor.

I am going to access your portacath. This will not hurt.

Voy a llevarlo a que le realicen una tomografía computarizada.

I am going to take you to get a CT scan.

Por favor, quédese quieto durante el procedimiento.
Este procedimiento no es doloroso.

Please stay still during the procedure. This procedure will not hurt.

Voy a llevarlo a que le tomen una imagen de resonancia magnética.

I am going to take you to get an MRI.

Por favor, quédese quieto durante el procedimiento.
Este procedimiento no es doloroso.

Please stay still during the procedure. This procedure will not hurt.

Voy a llevarlo a que le tomen una radiografía.

I am going to take you to get an X-ray.

Por favor, quédese quieto durante el procedimiento.
Este procedimiento no es doloroso.

Please stay still during the procedure. This procedure will not hurt.

Voy a llevarlo a la Unidad de Cuidados Intensivos (UCI).

I am going to take you to the Intensive Care Unit (ICU).

Voy a llevarlo a otra habitación.

I am going to take you to another room.

Voy a llevarlo de regreso a su habitación.

I am going to take you back to your room.

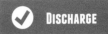
Photocopy this page.

Muchas gracias por haber venido hoy.
Thank you for seeing us today.

Por favor, llame al (_____) _____ – _____ **el día** ____ / ____
Please call _on_ **DÍA   MES**

para programar una cita de monitoreo para el día ____ / ____ / ____
to schedule a follow up appointment by **DÍA   MES   AÑO**

Puede obtener los medicamentos que le recetaron en:
You may fill your prescriptions at:

_____

El número de teléfono de ellos es:
Their phone number is: (_____) _____ – _____

La dirección de ellos es:
Their address is:

_____

Calle (Street)   **Apartamento** (Apt. #)

Ciudad (City)   **Estado** (State)   **Código Postal** (ZIP)

Si tiene preguntas sobre el seguro médico, por favor llame a:
If you have questions regarding medical insurance please call:

(_____) _____ – _____

COMMON NECESSITIES

148

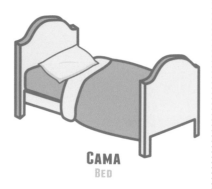

CAMA
BED

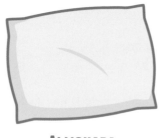

ALMOHADA
PILLOW

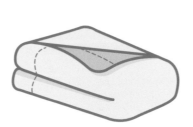

COBIJA
BLANKET

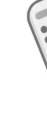

CONTROL REMOTO
TV REMOTE

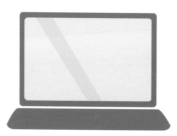

COMPUTADORA
COMPUTER

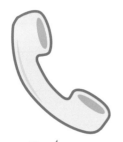

TELÉFONO
PHONE

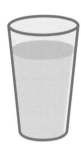

AGUA
WATER

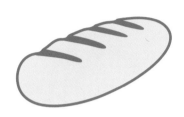

COMIDA
FOOD

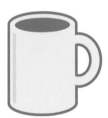

CAFÉ
COFFEE

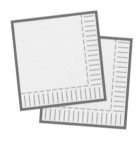

SERVILLETAS
NAPKINS

CUBIERTOS
SILVERWARE

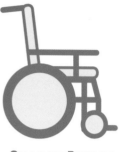

SILLA DE RUEDAS
WHEELCHAIR

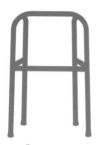

ANDADOR
WALKER

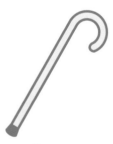

BASTON
CANE

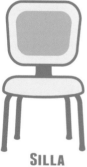

SILLA
CHAIR

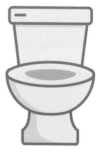

INODORO
TOILET

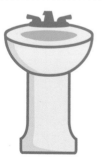

PILA
SINK

COMMON NECESSITIES

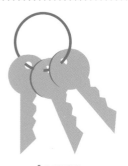

LLAVES
Keys

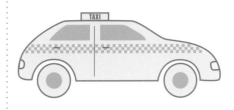

TAXI
Taxi

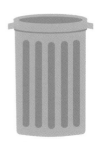

BASURERO
Trash Can

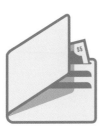

MONEDERO
Wallet

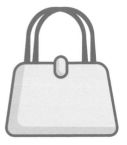

BOLSA
Purse

GAFAS
Glasses

ABOUT THE AUTHORS

Neil Bobenhouse, MHA, EMT-P

Neil Bobenhouse is a paramedic, entrepreneur, and language enthusiast formerly of the St. Louis City Fire Department. He holds a bachelor's degree in psychology and a master's degree in health administration, both from Saint Louis University. Neil founded Bobenhouse Industries with the vision to create real-world solutions for the healthcare industry.

Dean C. Meenach, RN, BSN, CEN, CCRN, CPEN, EMT-P

Dean Meenach has entered his 18th year of teaching and currently serves as Director of EMS Education/Paramedic Instructor and co-professor in the Paramedic to RN Bridge Program at Mineral Area College. He is a 22-year veteran in EMS and has served as a subject matter expert, author, national speaker, and collaborative author in micro-simulation programs. Dean continues to serve patients part-time as a member of a stroke team and in a pediatric and adult trauma center.

PHRASEBOOK CONTRIBUTORS

James A. Bobenhouse, MD
> Board Certified Neurology and Vascular Neurology
> Bryan Medical Center and St. Elizabeth Regional Medical Center
> Stroke Center Medical Director

Mark Levine, MD, FACEP
> Assistant Professor, Emergency Medicine
> Washington University School of Medicine
> Barnes-Jewish Hospital

Casey Regen, RN, TNCC

Morgan Grubbe, PT, DPT

All translations by International Institute of Saint Louis Language Services
Graphic Design & Illustrations by Andrea Molina
Previous Graphic Design & Illustrations by Ben Gathard

ACKNOWLEDGMENTS

The St. Louis City Fire Department
Washington University
Barnes-Jewish Hospital
Andrea Alameda, Shawn Bittle, Guy Jennings, Bhavin Mehta, Doug Randell, Matt Sleet, and Galen Taylor. Mike Barnes, Mike Beckenholdt, Jheree Coleman, Jack Douglas, Jeff Glorioso, Pam Miller, Ed Monser, Steve Ponzar, Dr. David Tan, Michelle Vaught, and Chris Yacula. Sarah Barekzai, Byron Beiermann, Stav Dor, Jake Flemming, Dr. Sai Iyer, Will Massanet, Laura Walsh, and Grace Pryor.